Child Protection for Hospital-based Practitioners

LOUISE HUMPHRIES MA, BA, RGN, RM, RHV
and
TIM GULLY BA (Hons), CQSW

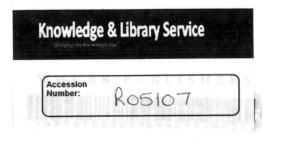

© 1999 Whurr Publishers
First published 1999 by
Whurr Publishers Ltd
19b Compton Terrace, London N1 2UN, England

British Library Cataloguing in Publication Data
A catalogue record for this book is available from the British
Library.

ISBN: 1 86156 102 4

Printed and bound in the UK by Athenaeum Press Ltd,
Gateshead, Tyne & Wear

Contents

Preface

This book is written to help medical and nursing staff, working within the Accident and Emergency departments and hospital-based sectors of the National Health (NHS), to understand the processes involved in child protection. However, it is highly relevant to all healthcare practitioners since it discusses the child protection process from initial concerns to potential legal involvement. It is written with the recognition that child protection is only one aspect of the work undertaken within the NHS and is intended to provide an overall grasp of the essential elements rather than a detailed account.

The text itself is written in as jargon free a style as possible and with the child's experience very much to the fore. Throughout the book there are a number of consistent themes combining legal framework, professional codes of conduct, practical application and the realities, benefits and difficulties often inherent in interagency working.

Language

The authors have attempted to balance the need for readability, clarity and accessibility with a desire to reflect the greater awareness that now exists amongst practitioners working with children and families for issues of gender, ethnicity, birth and disability. In the text, for consistency the terminology of the 1998 Children Act has been used; for instance the Act refers to all children as he. Rather than using the cumbersome parent/carer the single word 'parent' has been used to apply to all adults caring for children which should not be confused with the idea of parental responsibility.

Whenever quoting from the Children Act 1989 it is referred to as 'the Act'.

In all respects a child with a disability is a child first and disabled second with all the right to protection as his non-disabled peers. For this reason the authors have chosen not to make a special section for disabled children, deciding instead to use the word child as applying to all children. It is for the practitioner to adapt to any child's special needs, not for the child to be disadvantaged by any disability.

The Department of Health 1991 publication *Working Together Under the Children Act 1989* is referred to frequently throughout the book: to avoid unnecessary repetition following its first mention it is subsequently known as simply *Working Together*.

Introduction

This introduction is concerned with briefly placing child protection and therefore this book in context. The authors wish to assist the reader in gaining a greater appreciation of the issues and procedures current to child protection practice. It is hoped this will enhance the reader's own practice and contribute further to the work already undertaken daily to protect children. There will be no political statements or attempt to influence policy. However, the conclusion will discuss areas of possible reform, where practise in our opinion could be improved.

Child protection and child abuse are issues that affect all people whatever their job, experiences or training. Indeed one can argue that child protection is not simply the responsibility of certain organisations or practitioners, but the responsibility of everyone in society. It is often too easy to absolve ourselves of responsibility, expecting others to raise the concern or take action.

So, is writing a book on child protection a poor reflection on society? Does it make a statement about the way adults continue to treat and abuse children? Is it a sign of the times? It is understandable that one should want to place child protection in context with such questions. For many child abuse is simply unexplainable and a problem of unimaginable enormity. However, one can be positive that this is a society where the needs and rights of the child are more represented and protected than ever before. There have recently been significant developments with the introduction of the 1989 Children Act and an increasing understanding of working together as agencies in child protection.

Many of the changes began with concerns about health. Cholera, venereal disease, health and safety at work were all issues during the nineteenth century that provided impetus for change and more often than not the medical and nursing professions could be found supporting these campaigns, as it was these practitioners who saw the suffering at first hand. It is because of their unique position that health practitioners in hospitals and in the community have a vital role to play in child protection. Often it will be the practitioner in accident and emergency or on the ward, whom will first meet the victim, have to deal with injuries and the initial trauma and then focus on the possibility of child protection issues. The pressures at this stage cannot be underestimated, from the need to protect the child, the need to follow procedures and the need to deal with the family.

The issues and emotions entwined with child abuse can be distressing for all individuals, touching places that one hardly knew existed, or which have remained hidden. Some people have been victims of or witnessed abuse and understandably may find the abuse of children especially difficult to deal with at times. Practitioners would be less than human if working with children and families at such potentially traumatic times in their lives did not affect them, pulling them this way and that. One has to expect child abuse to trigger emotions in everyone that can add to the stress that may already exist.

It is important to remember that protecting children from abuse is only one aspect of the health practitioner's responsibility towards children, yet one that clearly fits into the overall services delivered to benefit the health and wellbeing of our children. In fact, much debate currently exists as to the practicalities of expanding the responsibilities of the already busy practitioner by adding the extra child protection responsibilities of the designated professional such as may be the case with the designated nurse, doctor or midwife. The underresourcing of child protection responsibilities and the expectation that these duties will somehow be accommodated can put the designated practitioner under a great deal of pressure. In turn, the practitioner seeking advice may have difficulty in obtaining the required information, or guidance in an acceptable time, as the designated practitioner may well be involved in other duties.

While recognising the operational difficulties that may exist, health involvement in child protection is essential. The British Paediatric Association has asserted that 'the purpose of health services for children is to enable as many children as possible to reach adulthood with their potential uncompromised by illness, environmental hazards or unhealthy lifestyle' (quoted in NHS Executive 1996, p. 6).

Health is one of the statutory agencies involved in child protection, and partly because of the Children Act 1989 is expected to work in partnership with the other agencies through formal policy-making bodies and operationally. The notion of partnership is used to inform our understanding of how practitioners should be working with families to promote the welfare of children, moving away from the traditional view that the practitioner knows best. Recent years have seen a significant step towards creating as comprehensive a system for child protection as is possible given the current climate and level of resourcing. These developments are located mainly within the last twenty years, perhaps beginning with the identification of the battered baby syndrome by the Kempes in the 1960s.

Developing working partnerships with children and families should be pivotal to our work and this book will address child protection based on issues within the wider family. It will not address at length stranger or paedophile abuse, but will place these briefly in context, i.e. that they are relatively rare and that practitioners need to be concentrating efforts on protecting children within the family. Organised and ritual abuse will be mentioned, but only when it occurs within the family; these issues are well catered for elsewhere.

This book is pulling the process together at a time of further significant change. There has been so much change in a short space of time and yet practitioners now face a period of further change, partly brought about by the political developments of 1997 and the lessons learned since the Children Act of 1989. New Labour have, after only two years in office, given clear indications that they wish to move the agenda once again and a new *Working Together* document is due for publication. The consultation document preparing the way for the new edition, entitled *Working Together to Safeguard our Children*, poses many questions which have arisen as a result of the lessons learned through current working practice and, sadly, the cases where things have gone wrong. Emphasis in the new document will be on working in partnership with vulnerable families towards prevention, reducing the need for reactive child protection intervention whilst retaining the need to act promptly when necessary. This is undoubtedly a commendable aim, but the conclusion will question the practical possibilities of this becoming a reality.

There are a number of ways in which the reader can use this book. It can be read from cover to cover, providing a clear, consistent and structured account of practice from the point of the identification of child abuse through the roles and responsibilities of the agencies involved, the process of the child protection conference and possible court involvement. Alternatively, the book can be used as a reminder of or introduction to specific areas of practice, for example the differences between family and criminal proceedings, or as a response to a reader's need for specific knowledge. In any event, the book will provide a useful reference and resource and prepare the ground for further reading according to need and interest.

The book also highlights the reality of situations, accepting that procedures are not always adhered to, that practices change from place to place and that conflict between organisations and between practitioners does exist. The text is strongly influenced by reality. It describes best practice within a procedural framework, whilst at the same time recognising the inherent difficulties that may emerge as a result of the various agencies' professional cultures and the strengths and weaknesses of the individuals involved. Organisations and human nature being what they are, protecting children is sometimes as much about balancing discordant elements as it is about keeping to procedures.

The most important thing is that throughout the child remains the focus; the child who, at times, during the heat of an investigation, is still all too easily forgotten.

Chapter 1
A historical perspective

Introduction

Today childhood is seen by most people as a special time, a period of life when children should be appropriately protected, allowed to thrive and grow, to develop physically, emotionally and intellectually free from danger and abuse. However, this has not always been the case and it is important to be aware of the development of our understanding of childhood and the child's position in society if practitioners are to fully appreciate why and how far they have progressed.

If history teaches nothing else, it demonstrates that child abuse in all its forms is not only a twentieth-century phenomenon. It has always and will always exist, both through omission and commission. It is possible to detect from nineteenth-century studies undertaken by such men as Charles Booth (*Life and Labour of the People in London*, 1889-1903), that children suffered abuse, physically, emotionally and through neglect. It is also apparent, from reading remarkably frank diaries, essays and letters written at the time by men whom would probably now be labelled as paedophiles, that child sexual abuse has also been a persistently identifiable element in British social history. What has changed is that practitioners have now come to recognise that these abuses exist and are developing evermore sophisticated methods of detection, management and treatment. This has been partly possible because practitioners now have a clearer understanding of a time called childhood.

It is fair to say that the way society thinks of children is a reflection of our time, which in turn is a reflection of our past. It is no longer appropriate, for instance, to send small children up chimneys, although child employment is still an active part of our society, often enhancing the child's developmental experience when appropriately

1

regulated and safeguarded. The debate around child employment in all its complexities and cultural perspectives is a current and lively one, and one that no doubt will affect the way society thinks of children and their role in the family and society in general. Sadly it is often the tragedies and extremes that challenge current thinking and encourage people to examine that which seems so normal as to be almost invisible. In our more enlightened society people may often take it for granted that things are now better for children than they were in the past, but, as Pollock and Maitlock (cited in Bainham and Cretney 1993) point out, too many professionals working with children still have to spend much of their time protecting children from intolerable situations rather than further improving tolerable situations for them. In order to understand this concept fully, one needs to consider where the concepts of child and childhood are located within society and what these may be. There is a need also to examine the relationship they occupy within the adult world of the law and the status of the child and view of the child from the legal perspective as it developed over time to the present day. The notion of parenting and the appropriateness of the care a child receives, the rights of a parent and child in relation to each other, the position children have occupied in society throughout the centuries are all concepts which are embodied within the way people think of children today. They have informed the current legislative framework in which practitioners are now required to practice.

These concepts will vary, not only in respect of time but also from within society itself as public awareness and understanding changes. Since the publication of the first broadsheets, public opinion has been influenced by the media as a result of high-profile cases often involving a child's death at the hands of those considered responsible for their care, protection and wellbeing. This may in turn stimulate judicial changes. Attitudes towards what is and is not socially acceptable change and have changed dramatically even during the course of the twentieth century. Until 1885 the age of consent was 13, incest did not become a criminal offence until early in the twentieth century, and history shows that child prostitution was a far greater problem in the past in terms of the actual number of children involved than it is today.

Childhood

The Norman Conquest and the introduction of Roman law provides a starting point with which to explore how people's understanding of childhood has evolved. Of this, the legal historian, lawyer, politician and judge Sir William Blackstone (1723-1780) wrote:

> The ancient Roman Law gave the father a power of life and death over his children; upon which the principle that he who gave has also the power to take away. Moreover a son could not acquire any property of his own during the life of his father, but all his acquisitions belonged to the father, or at least the profits of them for his life. (Blackstone, *Commentaries on the Laws of England*, Book 1, Chapter 15, Section 2, in Bainham and Cretney 1993, p. 9)

His words describe the absolute authority of the father and the subservient nature the child occupied in the relationship: no mention is made of the child's mother. The legal recognition of the supremacy of the father's authority over his domain, i.e. that of the family, extended to all aspects of the child's life and to all family matters. There is a need at this point to clarify that the socially constructed meaning of the word 'child' was very different to that of today. In order to understand this the practitioners need to consider the development of the concept of child together with the attendant implication to the child's experience during that period of life called 'childhood'.

Traditionally, when attempting to trace the development of the concept of child, the work of the historian Phillipe Aries has been a useful starting point. In his work *Centuries of Childhood* (1962), he locates the development of the concept of child and childhood within Europe in the sixteenth and seventeenth centuries, arguing that the development of this concept began within the more affluent middle classes of the time. The child, which would include an individual up to the age of around seven years, was seen as essentially innocent, untainted by the adult world which was seen as complex and corrupt by comparison. It is important to note that these concepts developed in the propertied classes. The life experience and expectations of the vast majority of children within the labouring poor would have been significantly different mainly due to the need for the child to work in order to increase the family's income, something that extended well into the nineteenth century.

Prior to this period, Aries argues that the concept of child and childhood did not exist to any significant extent. The child was only seen as such whilst needing the physical care and attention needed to survive. Once the child was no longer physically dependent, he was considered as part of the adult world and would be treated as such and included in adult activities. This would include sexual activities which, if seen from today's perspective and under the Act, would be considered as child sexual abuse.

Before the sixteenth and seventeenth centuries the legal view of the child was almost one of default in that the child itself was not a legal entity, only becoming so in terms of the father's property. Legal involvement at this time was mainly limited to issues of inheritance, in which the child was part of the property to be inherited. Legally the age of majority in the sixteenth century was defined as 'from the anniversary of the tenth birthday'; by the seventeenth century the age of majority had risen to 12.

The change in age at which childhood was at an end and adulthood begun was not based on any biological or psychological assessment of the child's development, but more from the social constructions of the day. Henry de Bracton, a leading medieval English jurist and author, identified that: 'In times past, girls and boys had soon attained the age [majority]: life was rude and there was not much to learn' (de Bracton c.1260). He argued that prolonging the disabilities and privileges of infancy during the medieval period resulted not from any growing understanding of childhood, but rather from the very practical introduction of heavy armour. The sons of kings (and members of the social elite) could only be regarded as 'full age' when strong enough to bear armour and to fight as knights.

The experience of children from the labouring poor would still have been associated with physical strength, but would have been significantly different to that of the social elite, with the age of majority probably younger and connected to the child's ability to take part in the labours of other family members. The child would have been expected to work alongside their parents or otherwise to contribute to the family income as soon as physically able. This in effect removed them at a very early age from the child's world, at which point they became small adults.

When considering the differing experience of childhood that existed within society, the experience in childhood of different genders is worthy of note. At this time the male could not marry until the age of 14 years, whilst it was commonplace for a female to be married and running a household, however that household was comprised, by the age of 10-12 years. The Marriage Act 1949 made a marriage void if under the age of 16 with parental consent under the age of 18. However if the marriage occurred without parental consent this in itself did not invalidate the marriage.

In association with the concept of the essential innocence of the child, Aries describes the emergence of a second concept of the child as a sort of adult plaything. The innocence of the child and their playful nature was seen as a source of amusement and entertain-

ment. This emergent concept developed as a result of the Reforma-
tion, the religious revolution of the sixteenth century that gave rise to
the various evangelical Protestant organisations of Christendom.
The child was, in this sense, seen as both innocent and untainted by
the corruption of the adult world with that essential innocence
putting them in need of a period of training and taming in order to
prepare them for the demands of adulthood. From the adult view-
point this period of time was seen as a preparation for adulthood
rather than a period for being a child.

In addition to those mentioned above there was a further concept
of childhood which began to emerge in the sixteenth century, originating in the teachings of John Calvin (1509-1564). Calvinism, as it
became known, saw the essential innocence of the child more in
terms of a risk of corruption to their mortal soul, a risk which, due to
their innocence they would be less able to resist and therefore would
put them at great spiritual peril. The child, unless trained, controlled
and disciplined by the father, was at risk of being condemned to a life
of sin and evil.

Again, it is worth noting that the experience of the vast majority
of children differed greatly from that of the social elite, a period of
training (education) and taming being unavailable to them due to
the requirement that they work in order to increase the family
income. This lack of a period of preparation and education amongst
the labouring poor furthered the view of the depravity of poverty as
seen from the perspective of the social elite - a view that can be
traced through the nineteenth century and into the twentieth.

The eighteenth century saw the development of the Methodist
movement of John Wesley (1703-1791), a result of which was that
childhood came to be seen as a period of innate depravity which,
unless driven from the child by discipline, control and absolute
obedience, would condemn the child to a life of sin and depravity.
The emphasis on the moral development of the child and the need
to physically drive out this innate depravity is characterised by the
expression 'spare the rod and spoil the child'. Indeed, it was seen as a
parental obligation to punish. It is difficult to say where the threshold
of justifiable and necessary punishment ended and child cruelty
began. It is, however, fare to say that the public threshold of the time
would have been considerably higher than today.

One of the common features of these schools of thought is the
view of the child (up to approximately seven years) as different from
the adult in respect of needs and abilities. The difference as
compared with the adult came to represent childhood. In other

words, children were children until they could physically take on the roles of their parents. This was an adult-centred as opposed to a child-centred view. Indeed, despite the fact that children had begun to be a distinct group within society, the legal view of children hardly changed in 800 years. This section began by quoting Blackstone on Roman law, and here it is interesting to quote him again on the child's position as he saw it at the time he was writing towards the end of the eighteenth century:

> The parent may lawfully correct his child, being under age, in a reasonable manner. For this is for the benefit of his education. The consent or concurrence of the parent (the father) to the marriage of the child under age, was also directed by our ancient law to be obtained ... and this is also a means which the law has put into the parents' hands in order to better discharge his duty; first of protecting his child from the snares of artful and designing persons and next, of settling property on his life, by preventing the ill consequences of too early and precipitate a marriage. A father has no other power over his son's estate, than as his trustee or guardian; for, though he may receive the profits during the child minority, yet he must account for them when he comes of age. He may indeed have the benefits of his child's labours while they live with him, and are maintained by him; but this is no more than he is entitled from his apprentice or servant. The legal power of the father (for the mother as such is entitled to no power, but only to reverence and respect) over the person of his children ceases at the age of 21 years: for they are then enfranchised by arriving at years of discretion, or that point at which the law has established (as some necessarily be established) when the empire of the father or other guardian gives place to the empire of reason. Yet until that age arrives, the empire of the father continues, even after his death; for he may by his will appoint a guardian to his children. He may also delegate part of his parental authority during his life to the tutor or schoolmaster of his child; who is then in *loco parentis* and has such a portion of the power the parent committed to his child, viz. that of restrain and correction, as may be necessary to answer the purpose for which he is employed. (Blackstone, *Commentaries on the Laws of England*, Book 1, Chapter 15, Section 2, in Bainham and Cretney 1993, p. 9)

Here the words of Blackstone describe the relationship between the adult and the child. He saw this in terms of the absolute authority of the father, or other as directed by him, over his child as subservient or apprentice, thus demonstrating the juxtaposition in relation to the current legal relationship between parent and child as one of the adult having responsibilities to rather than rights over the other. A point of note here is that this continued to be an underlying principle within the legal system until the Guardianship Act 1973 Social Services enacted that 'in relation to the legal custody or upbringing of a minor and in relation to his property or the application of income there from, a mother was to have the same rights and authority as the law had previously allowed the father' (S.1(i)).

The notion of the age of majority and the privilege of franchise was again limited to the social elite and the ability to exercise the right of franchise was given only to the property-owning male section of society. This continued to be the case until 1919 when non-property-owning males over 21 were, by act of Parliament, given the right of franchise and in 1919 when this right was extended to women over 30.

The absolute right of the father in relation to his family was unquestioned. The child, as such, was not seen as the bearer of any legal status except in relation to property ownership, inheritance and wardship, focusing on the child's property and inheritance rather than the child and his or her wellbeing. Thus it was unlikely that a child of the labouring poor would be subject to such legal considerations and as a result included within the legal construction or concept of child or childhood at that time. The legal construction was firmly located within the needs of the adult and as such dictated the social understanding of and expectations of children and the parent-child relationship. The right of the father also included the right to sell his child if he so chose to do.

In the event of the inheritance of property, the involvement of the law was from the perspective of the monarch as exercising absolute power over the subservient subject in the context of needing to protect the child from potential exploitation of an artful and devious adult. The child, as seen from the court, was unable to resist the manipulation of an artful adult, due to their relative immaturity, seen as a handicap as opposed to a developmental aspect of childhood. This legal construction resulted in the law preventing an adult from acting on a child's behalf in any legal matters, thus placing the child at some considerable disadvantage. (A point of interest here is that the death of Maria Caldwell at the hands of her mother's cohabitee in 1974 resulted in the creation of *guardian ad litem*, an officer appointed by the court to represent the interest of the child.) The only concession made by the court was to allow the presence of an adult as the child's 'next friend'. This remained the case until the seventeenth century when the child could appeal to the Court of Chancellery in order to be made a ward of court in respect of inheritance and the need for his maintenance until the age of majority. This relationship between the child and the law in terms of the care and protection a child received continued until the nineteenth century with the introduction of the Infant Life Protection Act 1872.

The child, although seen as being less able than the adult, was considered able to give unsworn evidence in court, unsworn if shown to be unable of understanding the nature of an oath. There was no blanket rule at which a child was considered able to give reliable evidence, the test of competency was left to the discretion of the presiding judge. The following quote from the scholar, judge and legal reformer Sir Matthew Hale (1609-1676) demonstrates this point, in which he describes the rape of a seven-year-old girl:

> If the rape be committed upon a child under 12 years, whether or not how she may be admitted to give evidence may be considerable. It seems to me that if it appears to the court, that she hath the sense and understanding that she knows and considers the obligation of an oath, though she be under 12 years she may be sworn. But if an infant of such tender years, that in point of discretion the court sees it unfit to swear her, yet I think she ought to be heard without an oath to give the court the information, thought singly of itself it ought not to move the jury to convict the offender, not with itself sufficient testimony, but because not on oath, without concurrence of the proofs, that may render the thing probable; and my reasons are:
>
> 1. The nature of the offence, which is most times secret, and no other testimony can be had of the doing of the fact, but the party upon whom it committed, though there may be other concurrent proofs of the fact when it is done.
> 2. Because if the child complains presently of the wrong doing to her mother or other relatives, their evidence upon oath shall be taken, yet it is but a narrative of which the child told them without oath, and holds much more reason of the child to hear the relation of the child herself than it second hand. (Hale 1993)

Revolution and reform

To gain identity in society an individual or group needs to have a value to those with power and influence; the greater the value the clearer the identity will be and the greater the associated protection and rights the individual and group will gather about them. Children during the 700 years following the Norman Conquest struggled to achieve a clearly defined identity, certainly outside of the elite where their value was measured in terms of social, political and military usefulness, for instance in terms of the first-born male inheriting land, titles etc. For the children of the labouring poor status was in terms of how much you could earn and this was an insubstantial status because life spans were brief and there were more where you came from. To change this situation there had to be dramatic socioeconomic changes, and they came in the form of a revolution.

This is not to say that individuals had not recognised the plight of children prior to this and tried to do something about it. Thomas

Coram was such an example. Between 1741 and his death in 1751, supported by wealthy benefactors, he organised the building of the first children's hospital in Great Britain, in Lamb's Conduit Fields in London. He had been moved to do so by the number of babies abandoned by their parents, left to die in the open. Thousands of children entered the hospital each year and the sheer demand eventually overwhelmed the venture. Individual actions could never be enough because it needed something far greater.

The industrial revolution that had begun hesitatingly during the eighteenth century in the mines and furnaces of Colebrookdale irrevocably changed the national economy from one based on a rich agricultural heritage to one dependant on urban industrial production. The pace of revolution accelerated unabated during the nineteenth century, bringing with it vast social and economic upheaval, none greater than the population shift from country to urban living. By 1851, for the first time, the towns contained more people than the country and, by 1881, over twice as many. For a country with a comparatively small population, 23 million at the time of the census in 1851 compared with France's 34 million, the impact cannot be underestimated. Yet, as Friedrich Engels suggests in *The Condition of the Working Class in England* (1849), this was a working-class movement brought about by the need for work and a naive if fatal optimism.

Families traded the unforgiving poverty of the countryside for the poverty, overcrowding, squalor and anonymity of the town. In small, country communities there had been a degree of identity and worth, however tenuous, but in the industrialised towns of nineteenth-century Britain people appeared to meld together providing a flow of labour that drove the machines to produce the wealth that fed and clothed the middle and upper classes.

> It contained several large streets all very like one another, and many small streets still more like one another, inhabited by people equally like one another, who all went in and out at the same hours, with the same sound upon the same pavements, to do the same work, and to whom every day was the same as yesterday and tomorrow, and every year the counterpart of the last and the next. (Dickens 1987, p. 22)

This was Charles Dickens' description of Coketown from *Hard Times* (1854), and it was the nearest many of his middle-class readers had come to the reality that existed in the industrialised towns. His vivid prose added to the reports contained in newspapers of child death, prostitution and neglect. Dickens was a propagandist and with the newspaper serialisation of such books as *Hard Times*, *Oliver Twist*, *Little Dorritt* and *Bleak House*, he fuelled the growing reforming attitudes of the new middle classes.

Urban families with more children than they could care for were left with stark choices. With no apparatus of state welfare to fall back on, families with little of substance had little alternative but to enter workhouses as brought to horrific life in *Oliver Twist*. Here was a society where human life was cheap, and no more so than that of a child. Industry quickly took advantage of this inexpensive and plentiful workforce, small enough to work in amongst the new, dangerous machinery. The attendant need for a large and inexpensive labour force in order to maximise production resulted in the increasing demand for child labour. The wages for child labour were considerably lower than that of an adult and at the same time represented a means of increasing the income of the vast majority of families. Child employment became an essential means of income and children were sent to work as soon as physically possible.

Yet infant mortality was high even amongst the wealthy, with women often dying in childbirth. The predominance of the paternalistic view informed Victorian thinking and thus the way the professions, the church and government viewed children and women. At all levels of society the new Victorian morality further reduced the child in status. By the end of the nineteenth century the child had become little more than the property of its parents, to be seen and not heard, and yet the reforming forces continued to erode old reactionary values and bring about change.

The increasing socioeconomic effects of the industrial revolution, together with the demands of the developing capitalist economy resulted, amongst other things, in an increasingly complex and demanding adult life. The expansion of the merchant classes, primarily in the textile industries, increased the need for the acquisition of academic skills amongst the middle classes. Levels of literacy increased and with it a desire to learn. There was more free time, a demand for information and a growing belief that things could be changed.

So here was something that could not have been predicted, that the industrial revolution would not simply be a revolution in technological terms, but an engine capable of changing the way people thought and acted. There had been a chain reaction. First, the new industries had sucked children in and vast wealth had been produced not only for the owners, but for the new middle management. The newly created middle class had found itself with time for leisure, to gain education, to read and think. Campaigners such as Wilberforce and writers such as Charles Dickens were there to stir up the issues upon which the reform movements could build.

The child as a visible part of society

This period of revolution and reform resulted in a significant change in the social relationship between children and adults. Whereas before children's role within the family had been taken for granted, during the nineteenth century children came to be defined more clearly as representing an economic status of their own; their visibility in society increased. Although still very much under the rule and control of the father, the child came to be seen socially as both an asset and a threat. The increasing economic status of the child changed the relationship between adult and child as society became increasingly dependent on the child to achieve economic prosperity. At this time the notion of the delinquent began to emerge and a new stage of childhood began. So began the concept of the 'troublesome teenage years' and the need for teenagers to be controlled and guided. For the first time, literature began to appear discussing the potential for unruly behaviour associated with this period of childhood. Activities with an emphasis on training and discipline developed, such as the Boys' Brigade. It is useful to note that the involvement of the police in family life at this time was considered appropriate to the management of a teenager who was seen as troublesome. If the father thought it necessary and with his consent, the police could remove a child to spend a night in a cell in order to instil a sense of self-discipline. This was in the absence of any actual or suspected criminal activity.

Arguably it was not until 1889 that the absolute rule of the father truly came to be questioned, when the law recognised the existence of the ill-treatment of a child by its parents as being a criminal offence by the introduction of the Prevention of Cruelty to and Protection of Children Act 1889. This recognition is seen as the beginning of the concept of the rights of a child to expect their parents to provide them with the care and protection now characteristic of the current legal framework some 100 years later. Indeed, prior to the 1889 Act there is some evidence that child stealing (considered to be child abduction in today's context) was used as a means of increased income by living off the child's earnings

As previously stated, the development of the concept of child and childhood as from a legal perspective is an extensive area of debate, and use of the available material has been necessarily limited as to be relevant within the context of this book. The law relating to adoption and divorce etc., although relevant to a certain extent, will not be considered to any great length within this discussion. However, this said, it would be useful to identify a point at which legal provision was made which, arguably, began the current inter-agency approach to the management of child protection and the development of the role of the police. This is worthy of note as, stated above, Roman law gave all rights to the father in respect of his family. It can be argued that the beginning of legal recognition of the need for children to be protected was the beginning of the recognition of the child as an individual as opposed to an extension of and property of the father.

Telford's Act, or the Custody of Infants Act 1839, allowed for the custody of a child to be awarded to the child's mother in preference to the father if necessary, provided that the child was under the age of seven years. This was later extended to 16 years by the Matrimonial Cases Act 1857, and the Custody of Infants Act 1873 recognised that a child may be in need of the court's protection in cases of parental separation. The wishes of the father are no longer the sole and driving consideration. The 1857 Act allowed the court to make such order as it considers appropriate in respect of the child.

The Guardianship of Infants Act 1886 removed the absolute right of the father to state in his will who the child's guardian would be in the event of his death. Prior to this the child could be removed from the family home irrespective of either the child's or their mother's wishes. For the first time, the 1886 Act allowed the court to consider the welfare of the child when deciding on such matters.

This legislation put in place the provision for the consideration of the welfare of the child to be the determining factor in court decision making, including the ability of the court to declare a parent to be unfit to care for their child. The absolute right of the father was further eroded by the Custody of Children Act 1891 by the provision of the court to refuse to allow for the removal of a child from where the child was living, if the court considered that the child had been previously abandoned there. The practice of abandoning young children to the care of such institutions as Dr Barnardos only to reclaim them once the child was physically able to work, and to provide the father with an income, was the driving force in the formulation of this provision. These legal changes demonstrate a significant change in the legal understanding of the relationship between parent and child by allowing the court to consider both the welfare and wishes of the child - a now familiar feature of the current legal framework.

With the turn of the century came an increasing public awareness of the subservient position of women in society in respect of the lack of women's suffrage, ownership of property, their status and access to the law, driven by the suffrage movement of which Emmeline Pankhurst (1858-1928) is traditionally seen as the principal advocate. The extent and effect on society of the women's suffrage movement was considerable and far reaching, and must, arguably, be born in mind when considering the social construction of children and the perceived appropriateness of the treatment and care they receive from adults.

The women's suffrage movement, later to become incorporated into the broader description of 'feminism', represents a significant school of thought much of which is beyond the scope of this book, however it had a direct effect on legislation in relation to children. The Guardianship of Infants Act 1925 was based on the principles of Sex Disqualification (Removal) Act 1919, as demonstrated by the following extract from the introduction to the 1925 Act:

> Whereas Parliament by the Sex Disqualification (Removal) Act 1919, its various other enactments, has sought to establish equality in law between the sexes, and it is expedient that this principle should obtain with respect of the guardianship of infants and the rights and responsibilities conferred by them.

The principle of state involvement in the provision of care for children was introduced by the Elizabethan poor laws of 1601. The responsibility of the state to intervene on behalf of a child considered destitute and/or abandoned was seen as an obligation of the state to provide for its vulnerable subject. This provision included the removal of a child from a family that was considered economically unable to support it, the economic consideration being considered as a legitimate reason for state intervention, removal and separation from the family. However, within these laws was the expectation that whilst the child had relatives the relatives would provide some assistance to the child even if the child was being cared for by the state. This concept of 'liable relative' was used to inform the Child Support Act 1991. Arguably then, the Elizabethan poor laws established the beginning of the principle that the child 'at risk' was a state responsibility and remained a responsibility of the family in the wider sense; a noticeable principle in today's legal framework is that the responsibility of the parents to their child is only removed by an adoption order, irrespective of other orders in relation to the child.

The practice of fostering pauper children during the 1800s resulted in the Poor Law Act of 1834. This Act transferred all rights in relation to the child from the parents to what was then called the Poor Law Union, responsible for overseeing the welfare of such children. Interestingly, much of the drive behind this change was the view that children are better placed within a family than within an institution such as the workhouse, where they risked becoming institutionalised and separate from society. The view that children tend to do better if placed with foster parents than if they live in a local authority children's home is a topical one in today's society, and one which informs statute policy and practice. The Poor Law Order of 1913 made it illegal for a child over the age of three years to remain in a workhouse for more than six weeks, and required the Poor Law Union to make suitable foster care arrangements.

In 1929 this responsibility was taken over by what is now the local authority, and represented a significant step towards current practice. The dissatisfaction and social unrest brought about by the Second World War at the care and management of orphaned and/or homeless children resulted in the appointment of a governmental committee. This committee was 'to enquire into existing methods of providing for children who, from loss of parent or from any case whatsoever, are deprived of a normal home life with their own parents or relatives; and to consider what further measures should be taken to ensure that these children are brought up under conditions best calculated to compensate them for parental care'. It was the report of this committee which lead to the Children Act 1948.

The emphasis of the 1948 Act to return children to the care of their parent as soon as possible resulted in some cases in a tendency of children requiring long-term care to drift within the care system without any long-term plans for the child's future whilst in care. As a result of this the Children Act 1975 allowed for the provision of parental responsibility to be transferred to the local authority in respect of a child who had been in care for more than three years.

The Children and Young Persons Act 1963 clearly identified the duty of the local authority to work with the services such as health and education in order to take all possible action either to prevent a child from appearing in front of a Juvenile court or from being received into care. The expectation of the services was that they would work together in the best interests of the child - an expectation common to all interagency work in today's setting.

Chapter 2
The legal
framework: the
Children Act 1989

Introduction

This chapter is designed to provide the reader with an insight into the legal framework in which they practice. Here will be considered the Act as it relates to child protection together with relevant government and professional guidance. It is important to note that this chapter should not be used in place of either practitioners' or legal advice where concerns over a child's safety or wellbeing may exist. In all such circumstances the reader is advised to discuss their concern with an appropriate colleague, i.e. a designated doctor or nurse. This should be done within a time frame which is not prejudicial to the child's safety or wellbeing. In circumstances where the risk to the child is considered to be immediate and it is not possible to contact the designated member of staff, the practitioner is advised to contact the relevant social services or police in accordance with local arrangements.

In all circumstances concerning a child's safety and wellbeing, the practitioner's primary responsibility is to act in the interest of the child and in accordance with the child's needs. Delay in taking appropriate action is only justifiable if it is clearly in the interests of the child.

The Children Act 1989

The principal legislative framework in which all medical and nursing staff practice is the Children Act (hereafter referred to as the Act), brought into effect in its entirety on 14 October 1991. The process that led directly to the Act began with the report of the House of Commons' Social Services Select Committee which was delivered to Parliament in 1984. It suggested that a thorough review of legislation relating to children was needed. Parliament agreed and the task fell to a DHSS working party that reported in the form of the Review of Child Care Law in 1985. Subsequently the government published a White Paper, *The Law on Child Care and Family Services*, in 1987. This became the basis of the Children Bill, which, with all-party support, began its passage through Parliament in November 1988 and received Royal assent in November 1989.

During the normal course of their duties it is not necessary for medical and nursing staff to have an in-depth knowledge as to the constitutional implications and impact of the Act or its application. However, an awareness of the change in legal emphasis, away from parental rights and to parental responsibility, will help the reader in understanding the fundamental change in the legal status of the child that has taken place. The child is now a bearer of rights, rights that are identified, protected and upheld in law, and the neglect of which by a parent is considered to be a criminal offence.

The Act was described by the then Lord Chancellor, Lord Mackay, as: 'The most comprehensive and far reaching reform of child law which has come before Parliament in living memory' *(Hansard (H.L.)* Vol 502, rol 488, 6 December 1988). His words were well chosen, as the Act introduced a number of underlying principles which represented a significant change in legal emphasis and understanding of the relationship between children and their parents. Perhaps most significantly, the Act changed the legal relationship between all parents and their children. It established parenthood as the primary legal status in relation to the child, introducing the concept of parental responsibility in the context of the parent's responsibilities to care for and protect the child in all matters until the child reaches the age of 18, a responsibility which can only be removed by an adoption order. (The interested reader should note that there may be variations to this depending on how parental responsibility is acquired, however for the purposes of this book the above is sufficient.) This principle replaces the previous understanding of the relationship between children and their parents based on parental rights. Thus the emphasis is now one of a parent's responsibilities to rather than rights over the child, which provides a child-centred focus - a consistent feature of the Act.

In addition to the introduction of parental responsibility (PR) the Act introduces the concept of partnership. Here it is clearly telling all those who work with children and their families that they must work in a manner that is open, honest and constructive, and to form a partnership with parents in providing the most effective means of care in order to promote the child's health and wellbeing. In most cases nursing and medical staff will have no difficulty in working in this way as the vast majority of the parents' wishes will be compatible with their child's needs. However, there will be occasions when the parents' wishes are not compatible with their child's needs, a situation in which the practitioner will require all their powers of support and persuasion in order to assist the parents to understand their child's needs and the consequences to the child if those needs are not met. Again, in the majority of cases, by following advice and support a solution will be reached which will meet both the needs of the child and the desire to work in partnership with the child's parents, thus achieving their support and understanding.

The Act does more than simply encourage partnership, it encourages non-intervention by the courts, placing the emphasis very much on the family and the agencies to work together in the best interests of the child. The Act creates several new private and public law orders, giving the court the widest choice of possibilities with which to meet the needs of the child, but it also insists that the court shall make no order unless it is better for the child to do so than to make no order at all. In each case the court has to ask itself the question: 'Do we need to make an order to safeguard the child's health and welfare?'

If the matter is to come to court then delay is seen as contrary to the interests of the child and to avoid this the court can control timing by using directions hearings in which formal agreement is reached about who are the parties, notice, filing and service of evidence and reports, and dates of future hearings. Expert witnesses need to inform the court of dates when they are available to carry out assessments and, later, to give evidence. The directions given may also cover the time available for an assessment or report, funding instructions, disclosure of information to experts, consent issues, venue of medical or psychiatric examinations, who will accompany a child, and the person(s) to whom the results should be given.

There will, however, be occasions when in spite of the efforts of all concerned or in circumstances where a child's injuries, for example, are inconsistent with the explanation provided, that the practitioner will be required to place the needs of the child over and above the desire to work in partnership with the family. In these circumstances the practitioner must act in the best interests of the child and in accordance with their own internal and Area Child Protection Committee (ACPC) policies and procedures. In such cases the practitioner will need to have a clear understanding of the relevant procedural guidance, an understanding which is best achieved in advance often within the context of an interagency training programme.

At this point it would be useful to consider the ways in which a child is or is likely to be at risk of suffering significant harm. Here it is helpful to look at the four categories in which a child's name can be recorded on a child protection register as taken from *Working Together Under the Children Act 1989* (DoH 1991).

- *Neglect*: The persistent or severe neglect of a child, or the failure to protect a child from exposure to any kind of danger, including cold or starvation, or extreme failure to carry out important aspects of care, resulting in the significant impairment of the child's health or development including non-organic failure to thrive.
- *Physical abuse*: Actual or risk of physical injury to a child, or failure to prevent physical injury (or suffering) to a child including deliberate poisoning, suffocation and Munchausen's syndrome by proxy.
- *Sexual abuse*: Actual or risk of sexual exploitation of a child or adolescent.
- *Emotional abuse*: Actual or risk of severe adverse effects on the emotional and behavioural development of a child caused by persistent or severe emotional ill-treatment or rejection.

Having introduced the above, it is important to note that at this stage the practitioner is not expected to make a judgement as to exactly which category the possible abuse may fit into, or whether their concerns would be sufficient to justify registration. These categories have been introduced to provide the reader with a reference point against which to balance their concerns and exercise their clinical judgement.

It is perhaps helpful to remind practitioners that the convening of a child protection conference and possible registration is not an inevitable consequence of the invoking of child protection procedures. It is, however, of vital importance that if a practitioner has concerns over the safety of a child these concerns are managed in a way in which the interests of the child remain the primary concern. The best way to do this is within the framework provided by both individual agency and interagency child protection procedures. The interagency approach to child protection procedures will be considered more fully in the following chapters.

As it is useful for the practitioner to be aware of the categories in which a child's name can be recorded, it is also useful to be aware of a second principle of the Act, known as the welfare principle. This requires a court to consider the welfare of the child as its paramount consideration, a consideration that will provide practitioners with a further reference point against which to balance their decisions and judgement. The following quote by Lord McDermott is worthy of inclusion as it ends sympathetically to the process of balancing judgements within a clinical setting:

> more than that the child's welfare is to be treated as the top item in a list of items relevant to the matter in question. [The words] connote a process whereby, when all the relevant facts, relationships, claims and wishes of the parents, risks, choices and other circumstances are taken into account and weighed, the course to be followed will be that which is most in the interests of the child's welfare as that term is now to be understood. That is the first consideration because it is of first importance and the paramount consideration because it rules upon or determines the course to be followed. (In Bainham and Cretney 1993, p. 43)

In coming to its decision, a court, in addition to applying the welfare principle, is also required to balance its decision against the welfare checklist. Again, this is introduced at this point to assist practitioners in exercising their judgement as to when to override the desire to work in partnership with parents when they do not consider the parents' wishes to be in the best interests of the child.

In addition, the Act requires that a court must consider what it describes as the welfare checklist in all its dealings and decision making regarding children. The Act requires the court to have regard in particular to:

(a) the ascertainable wishes and feelings of the child concerned (considered in the light of his age and understanding)
(b) his physical, emotional and educational needs
(c) the likely effect on him of any change in his circumstances
(d) his age, sex, background and any characteristics of his which the court considers relevant
(e) how capable each of his parents and any other person in relation to whom the court considers the question to be relevant is of meeting his needs
(f) the range of powers available to the court under the Act in the proceeding in question.

Clearly, the checklist described above is designed to be used within a courtroom setting. Within the clinical setting the practitioner will similarly be required to balance a number of issues in which the child's needs must be the central consideration.

In particular, parts (a) (b) (c) (d) and (e) are highly relevant to the clinical setting, with (f) perhaps applied to the course of action available to the practitioner, such as to contact the designated doctor or nurse, local social services and, if necessary, the police. At this point it is worth reminding ourselves that in circumstances where parental wishes may be in conflict with the needs of the child, support and a range of services can be offered by a more specialist practitioner in the field of child protection. These might include child protection social workers, specially trained police officers, health visitors and others who will work in partnership with parents to resolve this conflict, and the aim is to keep children within their families and cared for by their parents. In many circumstances this method of working is dependent upon the practitioner identifying a concern and acting appropriately. Not to do so may result in a child continuing to be at risk or continuing to suffer from significant harm. In addition to the above the practitioner can look to guidance from such documents as:

- Child Protection Guidance for Senior Nurses, Health Visitors and Midwives (DoH 1997)
- The Protection and Use of Patient Information (DoH 1996)
- Child Protection: Medical Responsibilities (DoH 1993)
- General Medical Council current advice
- Welfare of Children and Young People in Hospital (DoH 1991c)

Although not an exhaustive list, the above contain information relevant to this discussion and which practitioners may want to familiarise themselves. Advice issued by the General Medical Council provides that: 'Where a doctor believes that a patient may be the victim of abuse or neglect the patient's interests are paramount and will usually require the doctor to disclose information to an appropriate responsible person or officer of a statutory agency' (DoH 1993, p. 2). Here it is important to consider the pressures upon medical and nursing staff to maintain patient confidentiality. This is often an area which practitioners find the most difficult to balance: when is it acceptable to break the confidence of a patient and to disclose information entrusted in the context of the patient-practitioner relationship. There is no easy answer to this and will probably

Children Act checklist

Issue	Section
Paramountcy	Section 1 (1)
Delay	Section 1 (2)
No order principle	Section 1 (5)
Welfare checklist	Section 37
Emergency protection order	Section 44
Police protection	Section 46
Duty to investigate	Section 47

depend on many factors, not least of which is the confidence and understanding of the practitioner of the legal and interagency framework of child protection. However, the reader is reminded of the now numerous guidance documents which 'give permission' for confidentiality to be breached if the practitioner is doing so in order to promote or protect the welfare of a child they believe to be at risk.

Chapter 3
The statutory agencies: roles and responsibilities

Introduction

There is an assumption, not only amongst the public and the media, but also often amongst practitioners, that child protection is the sole and ultimate responsibility of the social services. While social services is certainly the agency that should take the lead in any child protection investigation, child protection is the responsibility of all agencies who have contact with children and their families.

The idea of working together, of interagency partnership and shared responsibility, is a relatively new one, and in child protection it can be the key to success or failure. The idea of sharing information with those outside immediate professional circles can cause concern as practitioners can no longer guarantee how it might be used. After all, as practitioners we know our immediate colleagues and how our own agency works, but may have only the vaguest notion about how our sister agencies are organised, operate and what they are likely to do with the information shared with them. Misconceptions and rumours may also exist and our own, or colleagues' 'bad experiences' may taint our view. This chapter contains a brief overview of what each of the other agencies involved in child protection actually do and how they contribute to the child protection process.

The central coordinating body that identifies and develops the strategic framework in which interagency child protection is managed is the Area Child Protection Committee (ACPC). *Working Together* identifies that:

> In every local authority area there is a need for a close working relationship between social services departments, the police service, medical practitioners, community health workers, the education sector and others who share a common aim to protect the child at risk. Co-operation at the individual case level needs to be supported by joint agency and management policies for child

protection, consistent with their policies and plans for related service provision. There needs to a recognised joint forum for developing, monitoring and reviewing child protection policies. This forum is the Area Child Protection Committee. (DoH 1991, Part 2, p. 5)

One of the main responsibilities of the ACPC is to produce an inter-agency child protection policy and procedures document which all agencies are expected to practise. It is a requirement that all agencies produce their own document that is commensurate to that of the ACPC's. This document should then be readily available to all practitioners who may be involved in child protection.

Social services

As described in Chapter 1, the Poor Law of 1834 services for children, the old, the infirm, the disabled and the young offender were administered locally by the Poor Law Union through the means of the workhouse as described by Charles Dickens in *Oliver Twist*. Throughout the nineteenth century and well into the twentieth, social need was seen as a result of poverty, sin and individual failure. As the nineteenth century progressed, the church and voluntary organisations such as the NSPCC began to supplement the work undertaken under the auspices of the Poor Law, but it was not until the 1940s that the system underwent real change.

In March 1945 the government set up a committee under the chairmanship of Dame Myra Curtis which proved to be a milestone in the development of services for children and families. It recommended that each responsible local authority should establish a children's department which would essentially unify services to children. However, services for other vulnerable groups in society remained fragmented. During the 1950s and 1960s social workers began to develop a shared identity whichever group in need they worked with and the traditional views of why people were in need began to be challenged with expanding research and literature.

It was not until 1971 that services for children, the elderly and people with disabilities were brought together within a single organisation. This came about following the publication of the Seebohm Report (1968) which was the decisive influence in producing the organisational structure of social services as exists in England and Wales today. In Scotland the Kilbrandon Report (1964) carried out a similar function. Seebohm espoused the development of generic social work teams and the 1970s saw authorities investing in a social services infrastructure with a clear managerial hierarchy and teams of qualified staff. However, in the light of a number of inquiries such as that concerning the death of Maria Caldwell, amongst other things, it became clear that the new organisation lacked a clear model by which to operate and needed to produce clearer procedures and develop interagency methods of working.

During the 1980s and 1990s, with further structural alterations, political changes and budget cuts, social services has struggled to find a clear identity and role in society. History may eventually demonstrate that it was the Act that finally cemented the role of the agency in place at least as far as children are concerned. Through this the organisation has responded positively in the area of child protection with the creation of clearer structures for interagency working and operational procedures. Social services departments have statutory responsibilities that, with child protection, make up a significant part of their core business, but the vast majority of resources go to those services delivered to the elderly. Through Care in the Community social services deliver many millions of pounds' worth of services that, whilst essential, provide a consistent drain on limited resources.

Today's social services will have offices in most towns, with workers in patch-based or specialist teams such as disability, services to the elderly, or children and families. The local department will also run family centres, homes for the elderly and children's homes. It is important to note here that the number of children accommodated by the local authority has dropped dramatically during the last decade, with the emphasis being placed on keeping the child within the family or with foster parents. As with health, many of these services may now be managed by the private sector.

As budgets have tightened, an increasing amount of the work undertaken by teams working with children and families is focused on child protection with little opportunity to undertake preventative interventions. However, with the imminent publication of a revised *Working Together* document this emphasis may change towards a preventative service based on family support. Support for this view has long been voiced and many would argue it was the basis of much work done prior to Seebohm; it is an issue examined in the conclusion.

Health

The following text contains a brief account of what may be of interest to the reader. It is a generic account, providing a minimum of information of some current and more recent issues. It does not focus entirely on the acute section of the NHS, but seeks to provide hospital-based practitioners with some of the more salient points likely to affect the community-based sector of the health service. Health authorities should be represented on the local ACPC and should appoint a senior doctor (usually the designated paediatrician), a senior designated nurse with a health-visiting qualification and a designated senior midwife to act as coordinators of all aspects of child protection work.

With the election of the Labour government in 1997 came the beginnings of significant changes for the NHS aimed at removing the purchaser, provider and internal market environment, replacing it with a system of integrated care. One of the principles upon which this is based is the need for a closer working relationship with local authorities, the minimisation of the internal organisational structures that inhibit communication across the various departments and a reduction in unnecessary bureaucracy.

With the introduction of healthcare based on national standards there is an emphasis on the role of the primary healthcare team (PHCT) and the need to develop closer working relationships between community- and hospital-based services. A commission for health improvement will be established, an independent body whose purpose will be to ensure a consistently high level of services at local level. With these changes is the emphasis on the improvement of public health and the prevention of ill health by addressing the damaging effects of issues such as poverty and deprivation.

The general practitioner (GP) has an essential part to play in child protection. It is likely that GPs will have known families for many years, perhaps for generations, and therefore has a unique picture of how they operate. They are well placed to make an early identification of child abuse or notice when a child may become vulnerable to, or experience significant harm. With their medical and social knowledge GPs can make a valuable contribution to conferences and long-term planning for the protection of the child. Amongst all their responsibilities to children and families, the GP's paramount responsibility is to the protection of the child.

It is essential that whenever a GP becomes aware that a child may be at risk of or experiencing abuse, these concerns be discussed with social services without delay. If there is clinical uncertainty then the GP should consult with colleagues, but even suspicions should be reported to social services as these may contribute to a wider picture being constructed on a family through interagency cooperation.

The police

The police force in England and Wales is based on a county structure and, apart from particular regional or national squads such as
the Obscene Publications Squad, issues of child protection are dealt
with at county level. As with each of the other agencies police
involvement in child protection comes at two levels; at a strategic
county or metropolitan level and operationally. At both of these their
primary responsibility is to protect the community and to bring
offenders to justice, but their overriding consideration is the welfare
of the child. However, in some circumstances the child's welfare may
be at odds with the demands of an investigation and possible prosecution of an offender. While the focus of police action will be to
determine whether a criminal offence has been committed and to
identify the person or persons responsible, it may not be in the interests of the child to secure the evidence to support the possibility of
criminal proceedings. (Chapter 6 looks at the issues surrounding the
gathering of evidence.) If this is the case the police may discontinue
with their investigation.

At county or metropolitan level senior police officers will attend
the ACPC and be involved in strategic planning of interagency child
protection. In addition they will involve the other child protection
agencies, in particular social services, in joint information sharing,
investigations and training. Under this umbrella it is at local level
that the police become directly involved with child protection, be it
through formal investigations following a disclosure or during their
day-to-day assignments. Many forces now encourage officers to be
aware of child protection and domestic violence in all their duties. In
this way not only can children be protected immediately, say with
formal police protection, but intelligence can also be gathered that
may contribute to future investigations.

The most likely beginning for police involvement comes following
a disclosure by a child. As the child's welfare must remain paramount it is vitally important that operationally initial discussions are
held between the police, social services and any other agency directly
involved with an alleged abuse to determine strategy as early in the
process as possible. This will mean that the child's needs will remain
a priority and that evidence, if required, can be collected in a way
that is systematic and child focused.

The decision for the police to withdraw from a child protection
investigation may come at several points during the process. It may
become apparent during the initial discussions that the child or

parents do not want the police involved and that this is felt appropriate, that there is not enough evidence to justify police involvement, or that it could be against the interests of the child for the police to remain involved. Although the police investigate allegations and gather evidence, it is the Crown Prosecution Service (CPS) which has the duty to examine the case and make the final decision on whether or not to conduct a criminal prosecution. If the police do continue with the investigation then the CPS decision whether or not proceedings should be initiated will be based on three main factors: whether or not there is sufficient evidence to prosecute; whether it is in the public interest that proceedings should be instigated against a particular offender; and whether or not it is in the interests of the child victim. In some cases discussions will be held between the police and the CPS prior to an investigation and/or during its course.

Even if the police decide after discussions with other agencies, and in particular social services, not to become directly involved in a child protection matter they can still provide an invaluable service by providing criminal histories and appropriate intelligence which can help the child protection investigation. The local police may be invited to conferences even if they have not been directly involved with the case.

The police have an emergency power that is not available to other agencies. Any police officer who has reasonable cause to believe that a child would otherwise be likely to suffer significant harm may remove the child, without prior application to a court, to suitable accommodation and keep the child there for up to 72 hours or ensure that he or she is not removed from hospital or any other place. This power may be used by the police acting alone, or in conjunction with social services or another child protection agency if speed is felt to be of the essence. The police can also obtain a warrant under Section 102 of the Act to enter premises and search for children. Again, where speed is essential to protect a child and a warrant could take too long to obtain the police can also enter premises in order to save life or prevent injury under Section 17(1)(e) of the Police and Criminal Evidence Act 1984.

Although the primary functions of the police, social services and other child protection agencies are different, one can see in the developing and cooperative relationship between the police and social services a genuine demonstration of the meaning of partnership in child protection. This does not mean that there are not problems in this relationship, but both the police and social services under the guidance of local ACPCs have worked to improve working methods and relationships. The difficulties that can be experienced in interagency joint investigations can be minimised through shared procedures, regular consultation and interagency training. The establishment of specialist child protection police units and specialist child protection teams or individuals within social services has helped to remove difficulties and enhance working together.

NSPCC

The NSPCC (National Society for the Prevention of Cruelty to Children) has a statutory duty to investigate cases of child abuse and has the power to convene conferences. This statutory role no longer fits easily with the present shape of the organisation. The NSPCC has during recent years dramatically changed its operational nature whilst maintaining its national image as an independent voluntary organisation representing the voice of children. The most significant of its recent achievements at a national level has been the national child protection helpline. The NSPCC is in fact a small organisation in terms of staff and many areas do not have a local NSPCC presence. Apart from the helpline, which is a communication point only, it is involved in little frontline child protection, concentrating its resources in post-abuse work, family support, assessments and work with adult sex offenders. The last element is a comparatively new departure and is seen as performing a preventative function. Each NSPCC project is in itself different, responding to local needs. Although a voluntary organisation well known for its fund raising schemes and street collections, the NSPCC is dependent on statutory funding for local operational direction.

Some NSPCC projects may in fact be 'staffed' by one individual performing an interagency coordination role, such as with adult sex offenders, or sitting as an independent chair for conferences. Projects will take referrals from children and families and from statutory agencies; where dependent on statutory funding the local project will be contracted to provide a specific service. Because of its flexibility the NSPCC is able to enable and manage innovative projects which can fill a gap in local services.

The NSPCC has projects in England, Ulster and Wales, but in Scotland the RSPCC (Royal Scottish Society for the Prevention of Cruelty to Children), performs a similar role and, like the NSPCC, works in consultation with the statutory agencies.

Education

The local authority education department will have a longer, continued contact with a single child or family of than most agencies. They
are also the only agency to have regular, ongoing involvement with
most children, although not with children educated in the independent (private or public) sector. (The private educational sector
creates issues that will be dealt with at the end of this section.)
Although education does not constitute an investigation or intervention service, the local authority education department should play a
key role in the child protection process, both in a statutory and
corporate sense and in a local operational sense.

The Department of Education Circular No 4/88, *Working Together
for the Protection of Children from Abuse Procedures Within the Educational
Service* (DoE 1988), recommends that schools designate a senior
member of staff, who may be the headteacher or another senior
member of staff, as having responsibility, under the procedures
established by the local education authority (LEA) for coordinating
action within the school. It also recommends that teachers should be
alert to signs of abuse and that designating one teacher with a special
responsibility for child protection does not remove the responsibility
of all school staff to be aware of such signs. Because of their day-to-
day contact with a child, school staff are particularly well placed to
observe outward signs of abuse and changes in behaviour. The
Circular states that in all cases where a teacher or other member of
the school staff has good cause to be concerned about the welfare of
a child, they should report their concerns to the designated member
of staff.

Headteachers and teachers with particular knowledge of a child
or family will be involved in the child protection process and may be
invited to attend conferences. As well as regular members of school
staff there will be other specialist practitioners visiting school
premises and becoming involved with the staff and children. The
ones mentioned here are those most likely to become involved in
child protection matters and to attend conferences.

LEAs will employ teams of education welfare officers (EWOs) or
education social workers. Each school will have an allocated welfare
officer and each officer is likely to have more than one school, possibly a secondary and the primary and middle schools in the catch-
ment area. It is the task of the welfare officer to ensure that children
get the maximum benefit from the educational facilities available.
Anything that could affect a child attending school or encourage a

child to truant comes within their remit; this may include bullying, child abuse, family problems or ill health.

The educational psychologist, employed by the psychological service of the LEA, can provide help by direct involvement with children and through advice and work with adults in regular contact with children. In local authority schools there may be be a school nurse employed by the district health authority or trust. They will make regular visits to schools and are permanently attached to most special needs schools. They can play an important role in the detection and prevention of child abuse.

Independent schools are not obliged to have child protection procedures and, unless children are boarding at the school, the local authority has no power to inspect. Independent schools are encouraged to liaise with the ACPC and social services to share knowledge and skills, but this can depend on local arrangements. Often independent schools will have a significant number of non-UK students or students from a wide area and this can create further difficulties in contacting parents who may, for instance, be abroad.

Probation service

The probation service usually begins its work with an offender when either the magistrates' or Crown Court requests a report. This will be prepared by a probation officer and will include details of the offender's background, circumstances and the sentencing options open to the court. When the court orders a period of probation, the offender is placed under the supervision of a probation officer, with the conditions of probation specified by the court, which may require the offender to attend a management programme. Such programmes have become common and may include work with anger management, drugs and alcohol misuse and sex offending.

The court may order a period of community service that is also supervised by the probation service, or impose a custodial sentence. The probation service has traditionally worked in prisons, providing a link to the community for the inmates, but also playing an active part in parole adjudications and release plans. Upon release from prison the offender will often be supervised by a probation officer who will liaise with colleagues from other agencies as and when necessary.

Over recent years the probation service in England, Wales and Northern Ireland has changed in character from a service that set out to inhibit offending by 'befriending' and working alongside a wide range of individual offenders, to an organisation providing community-based sentences for the more severe and persistent offender. In general, its role in child protection now centres on its knowledge of the offender. This focus, while narrow, can be used to great effect in interagency planning for child protection, offender supervision and treatment. There are now a significant number of interagency projects throughout England and Wales where the probation service, social services and the NSPCC have come together to work with adult sex offenders. This allows the victim's view to be represented and many would argue that it is essential for such a project to be interagency to be effective.

Other agencies

It is important to bear in mind that the voluntary sector and armed services have a significant and relevant role to play, the extent of which may vary according to area. For instance, if an area has a significant number of military personnel living within its boundary then the particular service, or services, may be represented on the ACPC and attend conferences. The particular armed service involved will seek to cooperate with statutory agencies and support service families where child abuse is suspected or has occurred. As with any agency involved in the process they hold information that can be essential to protecting a child successfully, or assist in the assessment and review process. There is also the Soldiers, Sailors, Airmen Families Association (SSAFA), which provides a social work service to children and families living abroad.

In addition, the local authority housing departments and housing associations, together with other relevant groups such as domestic violence forums, need to be incorporated within the ACPC framework. Indeed, any voluntary organisation working with children, such as the Boys' Brigade and Scouting movement, may call upon the ACPC for assistance and guidance in developing their own child protection procedures and improving links with child protection agencies.

Chapter 4
The child protection process

Introduction

This chapter provides the reader with an account of what to do when faced with a situation concerning a child's safety. It includes a discussion of the professionals likely to be involved and their role in the interagency child protection process. Child protection concerns can arise in many circumstances, for example, when a child is seen in the accident and emergency (A&E) department, on the ward, as an inpatient, outpatient, or as a visitor, or when he or she is the child of a patient or, indeed, unborn. All of these are situations in which hospital staff may become concerned that a child is at risk. During the course of the discussion, guidance provided by the British Medical Association and the role of the consultant paediatrician and other medical personnel will be considered.

The discussion is first in relation to child abuse in general and best practice issues, before considering child sexual abuse. The reason for this separation is that child sexual abuse has a number of specific considerations which the healthcare practitioner has to be aware of. In addition, the identification and management of suspected child sexual abuse has often been described as the area of child protection that causes practitioners most concern. In conclusion there is a brief discussion of situations in which an allegation is made against a member of staff.

By its nature, the discussion is highly process-orientated and the reader is reminded to ensure they have a good working knowledge of the child protection procedures as relevant to their place of work. These may vary in accordance with local arrangements.

It is also worth emphasising at this point that the following of procedures alone will not provide the reader with the depth of understanding achieved by participation in interagency training, the benefit of which leads to a greater level of understanding of the roles and responsibilities of the agencies involved and the development of practitioner networking, which in turn leads to a greater level of protection for the child population.

The accident and emergency department

Childhood is a time in human lives when we learn about the environment in which we live, learning which often occurs without the benefit of a sense of danger and caution that comes with experience. The child is destined to explore, test and challenge and, as a result, will have accidents. This may sound like 'common sense' and is probably true in most cases. However, as practitioners charged with maintaining the interest of the child as the paramount consideration in all work that brings them into contact with children, there is a need to look into this just a little more closely. Children must be allowed the freedom to develop, indeed not to do so can, in some circumstances be considered as abuse; however, the adults responsible for their care must also protect children from unnecessary exposure to danger.

The difficulties facing the practitioner in the A&E department when trying to assess whether a child's injury or condition is developmentally appropriate, if the given explanation is likely or if the demeanours of the child and his or her parents are 'appropriate', for example, can be considerable. Good practice suggests that in most cases practitioners are unlikely to be faced with a situation where child abuse is clearly the most likely explanation, although this may of course happen. In most cases the practitioner is more likely to suspect or feel uneasy, and it is in these circumstances where there is a risk of practitioners convincing themselves that they must be wrong, as no one is comfortable with the thought that a child's injuries or condition could have been inflicted either intentionally or through neglect. These is no simple solution to this dilemma but to remind ourselves always to think the unthinkable and to take anything the child may say seriously, should the child say something which causes concern, as not to do so could mean that a child is put at further risk. Here exists a second dilemma in that, as described above, children will have accidents and will become ill from time to time and those charged with their care will sometimes look to nursing and medical staff as a source of help. Fear that they will be accused of abusing or neglecting their child is often a very real anxiety felt by parents who need to be reassured that a visit to A&E does not automatically lead to a conference and the removal of their child. Media portrayals of 'newsworthy cases', which by their nature are sadly associated with the most serious cases of abuse to children, can do little to reassure the anxious parent. The reality that even if abuse is suspected it is by no means automatic that a conference will be necessary and even less likely that the child will be removed is rarely the public's perception. Therefore the professional is faced with the difficult task of balancing support and reassurance of the child's parents whilst having to think the unthinkable in order to disregard it as a possible explanation if appropriate to do so. The Act confirms that in all circumstances it is the child's welfare that must be upper-most in the practitioner's mind. In order to help practitioners all hospitals should have clearly defined child protection procedures, the following of which is in the interest all concerned. It is recommended that all staff who are likely to have contact with children have an appropriate level of child protection training and are fully aware of the information contained in the child protection procedures.

When presenting at an A&E department it is good practice for a child to be allocated to a named qualified nurse and to have a full history taken, including, for example, any delay in seeking advice, the explanation given, previous attendance at A&E and an account of how the injury/condition arose. The child should undergo a thor-ough medical examination as appropriate to his or her condition and as consistent with normal practice, bearing in mind that children under the age of five are at highest risk of physical abuse and should therefore be undressed and examined. Should the practitioner become concerned, the action taken will largely depend on the circumstances. It is advisable to discuss any concerns with the child's consultant paediatrician, designated doctor or nurse admitting the child if necessary. If the situation arises where concerns exist and the parents refuse to allow the child to be admitted then emergency action may need to be taken and the relevant social services depart-ment contacted (or the emergency duty team if out of hours or the police in accordance with local arrangements). If following discussion the level of risk is not thought to warrant admission then prompt liai-son should take place between the appropriate member of the hospi-tal staff, the child's health visitor/school nurse, the midwife if the child is unborn or still under the care of a midwife, and the GP. A prompt referral should be made to the relevant social services depart-ment clearly stating the concerns and that this is considered to be a child protection referral. Record keeping and making a referral to the social services will be discussed in more detail in the following text.

The child on the ward

If a child has been admitted, his care should be allocated to a qualified, named nurse who should take responsibility for ensuring that effective communication takes place between all those involved with the child's care, community-based staff and the relevant social services department. The designated doctor and nurse will often also take responsibility for inter- and intra-agency communication in accordance with local arrangements. Careful and detailed records should be kept by all concerned, distinguishing between matters which are directly observed or reported. All entries should be timed, dated and signed and include an account of any decisions made and the reasons for those decisions. It is the responsibility of all professionals to ensure that a prompt referral is made to the relevant social services department, even in the event of disagreement. Should disagreement arise, further discussion with the designated doctor and nurse is advisable.

Once the relevant social services department has been informed, it is their responsibility to undertake a child protection investigation and, if appropriate, nursing and medical staff have a duty to assist them and to share information on a need-to-know basis. It will assist social services greatly if nursing and medical staff clearly identify their concerns together with their reason, stating that they consider this to be a child protection referral.

Once social services have become involved, whether the child is an inpatient or living in the community, they will, if it is felt appropriate, undertake a child protection investigation in accordance with Section 47 of the Act. This investigation will involve liaison with relevant agencies and often a discussion with the police. During the course of the investigation social services will decide if it is appropriate to continue to a conference. The decision of social services to contact the parents will depend on the information they have - if the decision is made that a conference is necessary the parent will be contacted and involved. It may be that social services, upon liaison with other agencies, find that no further action is necessary, in which case they may or may not involve the child's parents. It may also be that upon liaison with other agencies social services find that the child and his or her parents can more appropriately be supported in ways other than child protection, for example as a child in need in accordance with Section 17 of the Act or, possibly, Section 11. Nursing and medical staff should take advice from social services as to the planned management of the investigation that may involve their attendance at strategy meetings and possibly the provision of a report. It is important to note that this investigation must take place within eight days, with the decision to contact the child's parents being made very early on in the process. (A greater explanation of the process of a Section 47 investigation can be found in Chapters 7 and 8.) It is worth remembering that a referral to social services which, following investigation, does not continue to a conference is not an inappropriate referral and should not discourage contact with the social services in the future. The vast majority of children referred to social services as children at risk are supported in ways other than by the use of Section 47 of the Act. However, the level of risk facing a child must be assessed before a decision can be made as to the most appropriate means of protection and support.

Child protection medical responsibilities

If a child is admitted where concerns for that child's safety exist, or if concerns arise during the course of their admission, or if they are seen in the A&E department, medical staff should discuss their concerns with the relevant consultant paediatrician, either the consultant on call for the day or the designated doctor. If a child's care is the responsibility of a medical or surgical team other than paediatrics and child protection concerns exist, it is the consultant paediatrician who has responsibility for the child protection aspect in all cases involving a child protection concern irrespective of the discipline of the team which has responsibility for the child's care. The child protection procedures should be followed, taking into account the need for a careful history in addition to that which would normally be taken as a result of the child's condition. Other examinations include a developmental assessment with the use of centiles, radiological skeletal surveys, blood-clotting screens, written opinion of the specialist consultant - such as orthopaedic, neurological etc. - and the collation of records, including those of siblings.

When consulting with the social services, medical staff should be prepared to give an opinion as to whether the child's injury/condition is likely to have been caused by abuse and/or neglect. It is important that medical staff provide social services with clear information to assist them to undertake their child protection duties in as effective manner as possible.

Should a parent attempt to remove a child who has either been admitted from the A&E department as a result of concerns, admitted from the community as a result of concerns or where concerns have arisen during any other method of admission, immediate advice must be sought from the relevant designated nurse, doctor, social services department, emergency duty team or police, as appropriate and in accordance with local arrangements.

It may be that the social services apply to the local magistrates' court (families panel) for an emergency protection order (EPO), or perhaps a prohibitive steps order, to maintain the child on the ward. Should this happen it is possible that nursing and medical staff will be asked to provide the court with a statement or be required to attend in person. In these circumstances advice should be sought from the designated doctor or nurse and possibly a legal representative. Professional organisations are a further source of advice.

Child sexual abuse

Having discussed the responsibilities of health practitioners in relation to physical and emotional abuse and neglect, this section discusses those responsibilities where child sexual abuse is the concern. The reason for considering this type of child abuse separately is that it is often identified by those whose work brings them into contact with children as the area of abuse which causes them the highest level of anxiety. As with other forms of abuse, the child protection procedures should be followed in all circumstances and the practitioner is reminded to 'think the unthinkable'. However, unlike other forms of abuse sexual abuse will rarely have 'medical' indications, the diagnosis more usually being made by a combination of social factors such as the child's demeanour, behaviour, performance at school and possibly a disclosure. This is not to say that children who have been physically or emotionally abused or neglected do not demonstrate their abuse in their behaviour or that they may not disclose their abuse, as they may well do. However, the role of medical and nursing staff in protecting a child in these circumstances does vary slightly.

If a child should present with clinical features which suggest he or she has been sexually abused the practitioner concerned should not undertake an examination in this respect unless specifically trained to do so for a number of reasons. Those who are specifically trained, such as police surgeons, will undertake the examination in such a way as to allow their findings to be admissible as evidence should court proceeding result. However, it is advisable to remember that all records can be used as evidence should a court so direct, not only those taken for that specific purpose (see Chapters 6 and 9). The need for a child to be examined more than once should always be avoided. If an untrained professional examines the child and evidence is needed for court proceedings, the child may need to be examined a second time. Child sexual abuse can be difficult to diagnose clinically, although occasionally definite diagnoses can be made by, for example, the presence of seminal fluid in a child's anus.

Having said this, practitioners are far more likely to become concerned by means other than direct medical evidence and should act in accordance with their concerns and the relevant child protection procedures as described above.

Should a child say something that causes a practitioner to be concerned, whatever the type of abuse, the child should be listened to and what is said taken seriously. The practitioner should reassure him that it is okay to tell, not attempt to question a child or attempt to stop him from talking. It is important that the child is not promised absolute confidentiality, as this information must be shared with those who need to know in order to help him. The practitioner should make a careful note of what the child says. If, following a child protection referral and as part of a Section 47 investigation, it is considered appropriate and necessary to interview the child it will be done by specially trained personnel. Should the child be interviewed for evidential purposes it will be done in accordance with the Home Office/Department of Health publication *The Memorandum of Good Practice* (Home Office/DoH 1992) and will be undertaken by a specifically trained social worker and police officer working as a team. This will be discussed more fully in the following chapters.

Allegations of abuse involving members of staff

If an allegation of abuse is made against any member of staff, that allegation must be taken seriously. Child protection procedures should identify the possibility of abuse by staff and provide a process by which such allegations are to be managed. This process should be produced in discussion with personnel, management, unions and professional bodies and should take into account professional, non-professional and voluntary staff. In addition, there should be the recognition that an allegation may be made against a member of staff and following investigation be found to be untrue.

If any member of staff receives an allegation or becomes concerned that a member of staff may be abusing a child (or children) they must take this concern to an identified senior member of staff according to local arrangements. This member of staff should immediately discuss the concerns with the relevant social services department. There may be an identified member of staff to contact in these circumstances. In many areas the chair of the ACPC should also be informed.

It may be that a strategy meeting will take place involving police, social services and hospital staff. Any decision to discuss the allegation with the member of staff concerned will often be taken at this meeting together with the process of investigation, the need to suspend the member of staff (without prejudice) and the support which is to be offered to them during the course of the investigation. Once the outcome of the investigation is known, the appropriate decisions can be made as to reinstating the member of staff or, if appropriate, initiating disciplinary and possibly criminal proceedings.

There is also an understandable fear that children may make false allegations against members of staff, possibly during examination or treatment. This is a rare occurrence and staff should follow good practice guidelines.

Chapter 5
The identification of child abuse

Introduction

This chapter takes the reader through the four categories of abuse as described in the Department of Health document *Working Together*. It is against one or more of these categories that a child's name can be recorded on the child protection register (CPR) if, following a child protection investigation by the social services and possibly the police a conference decides that the child has either suffered from or is at risk of suffering from significant harm.

It is the social services who have a duty to investigate under the Act if they have reason to believe that a child living in their area is either suffering from or is likely to suffer from significant harm. The purpose of this investigation is to decide if a conference should be convened. This will be in consultation with the agencies involved with the child and his or her family, together with the child and the family themselves. As shall be demonstrated in detail in Chapter 7, representatives from the relevant agencies will be invited to attend, as are the parents and child if appropriate. The purposes of a conference is to provide an interagency forum in which concerns relating to a child's safety and wellbeing can be discussed and, having done so, in which decisions can be taken as to whether those concerns constitute significant harm to the child. If so, the next decision will be to decide which of the four categories best describes the nature of that significant harm and record the child's name on the CPR. One or more categories may be used according to the definition. Should a child's name be recorded, the next step will be to identify an inter-agency plan to protect the child with a view to removing or minimising the risk and therefore remove his name from the CPR.

It is the child protection plan rather than the registration of the child's name that provides the child with protection. The registration acts as an indicator to highlight the risk status of the child. In the majority of cases children are protected within their own homes, with the agencies working with the child's parents to achieve a positive outcome for the child concerned. The progress made by the child's family is reviewed at a review conference held no later than six months after the date of recording the child's name. Should the progress be sufficient to reduce the risk to the child, the child's name will be deregistered. If further work is considered necessary this will be undertaken and again reviewed at a subsequent review conference in no later than six months.

At the point of initial concern the responsibility of practitioners is to undertake their normal duties in respect of the care they would provide for the child and their parents and, in addition, to place the child's safety as their primary and overriding concern and share those concerns with the designated doctor, nurse or midwife as appropriate. The speed at which this is to be done will largely depend on the child's circumstances. However, it should be undertaken in a timely manner with a minimum of delay. Once those concerns have been shared, those who specialise in child protection will in discussion with the practitioner decide on the next course of action.

The decision to proceed to a child protection investigation and possible conference is not an inevitable one. However, the protection of a child is dependent on timely and appropriate action by all concerned. To help the practitioner in deciding if the concerns they have are significant, it is useful to look at the definition of significant harm as provided in the Act. In addition it is helpful to keep in mind that harm can be significant to a child either in the seriousness of its effect or by its implication. For example, a child may present at the A&E with a minor injury, but if that injury was sustained as a result of an unrealistic expectation of the child's developmental ability to protect himself and anticipate the consequences of his actions, the contextual effect of the child's lifestyle may well constitute a risk of significant harm. Therefore it is important to keep in mind that the categories of abuse under which a child's name can be registered and the definition of significant harm is the standard applied as an end product. It should not be used as a standard by which to decide whether or not to share a concern.

The process of a child protection investigation and possible conference will not be discussed in this chapter but will be covered in detail in Chapters 6, 7 and 8. The following discussion considers the context in which a child may be 'at risk'. It will not be a list of signs and symptoms as this approach carries a danger of presenting a checklist of possible concerns. Significant harm to a child is a complex 'diagnosis' and cannot be minimised to fit easily within such an approach. The danger in so doing is to suggest 'yes' or 'no' answers to a concern which is more usually and appropriately answered within the holistic experience of the child.

It is useful to remember at this stage that a risk of significant harm can also include the unborn child. Concerns in this context are most likely to be voiced if the mother and/or father has a previous history of child abuse, or when the pregnant mother is abusing herself, or is herself at risk of domestic violence from a partner, in such a way that the unborn or newborn baby will be at risk. If a mother or father is suffering from a mental illness that may restrict their ability to care for the child after birth then a conference may be convened and the child's name may be recorded on the CPR. In addition, in the case of a mother who is unable to care for herself during pregnancy and as a result places her unborn child at risk a conference may be convened. In these circumstances the process is the same: the practitioner should share those concerns with the designated doctor, nurse or midwife according to local arrangements.

It is fair to say that a considerable amount of material has been written in relation to the identification of child abuse, often with each of the categories of abuse constituting many publications in their own right. Coverage in this chapter is limited and will focus on the minimum needed by hospital-based practitioners whose work may bring them into contact with children and their families. The discussion will focus on the abuse of children by family members rather than by other adults the child may come into contact with such as teachers, neighbours, an activity leader or, very unusually, a stranger. In addition, the discussion will not include issues to do with the abuse of a child or young person by another child or young person. The interested reader is advised to refer to the bibliography for further information.

Significant harm

The notion of significant harm is a central tenet to the Act and the process of interagency child protection, and one which can at times seem a difficult concept to demonstrate. Practitioners may find themselves questioning their own values and whether or not they are inappropriately transferring those values to a child and his family. A general rule to keep in mind is that harm is harm however it has been caused in whatever setting. When faced with a concern, contrast what would be expected of a similar child against the issues of concern; if the concern remains then it is reasonable to consider that the concern could demonstrate significant harm.

The Act defines significant harm as follows:

- *harm* means ill treatment or the impairment of health or development
- *development* means physical, intellectual, emotional, social or behavioural development
- *health* means physical or mental health
- *ill-treatment* includes sexual abuse and forms of ill treatment which are not physical.

> Where the question of harm suffered by a child is significant in terms of the child's health or development, his health or development shall be compared with that which could reasonably be expected of a similar child. (Children Act 1989, S.31(10))

The above definition is broad and allows the various practitioners whose work brings them into contact with children and their families to exercise their judgement and expertise.

At this point it is important to mention the concept of secondary significant harm. This may be considered when a child has no injuries, evidence of sexual assault or neglect and no apparent harm from emotional abuse. It may also be useful alongside an identifiable abuse to assist in broadening the picture of the environment and circumstances in which a particular child lives. It can be argued that a child growing up in certain situations may suffer from exposure to beliefs and behaviours in the adults caring for them that will impact negatively upon that child's thinking, attitudes and behaviour. For instance, a child may learn from a father to have inappropriate views of women which the child may replicate in his future life. Domestic violence need not be physical, or obviously verbally aggressive, but can be subtle with no obvious primary impact upon the child, yet the secondary harm that child may suffer can be significant.

Harm, therefore, can be serious in itself by the effect it has on the child directly and by possible complications which may arise as a result of it: its cumulative effect or by its implication. It is worth spending time to unpack this a little more as the notion of significant harm can be a difficult one with which to grapple. There will be situations where the experience a child has is clearly harmful, such as the child whose parent, for whatever reason, fails to respond to an anticipated danger - for example preventing a three-year-old from climbing out of a window from which the child then falls and sustains an injury as a result. In this example the harm experienced by the child has been caused, strictly speaking, as a result of the injury.

The context is all-important when assessing the holistic experience that a child has of childhood. Without the health visitor, who could provide the benefit of other information such as, for example, the home circumstances and general level of care, practitioners must act on what is 'in front of them', taking into account the explanation of how the injury/illness occurred and the attitude of the child and parents. In this case the child could be well cared for, well protected and no more at risk of harm than any child would be simply as a result of being a child. However, the child may have a childhood experience of neglect and be at considerable risk of that harm being significant due to the cumulative effects of poor or inadequate parenting.

Practitioners can be faced with a far from obvious picture, often dependent on what the parents are saying. It is fair to say that practitioners are trained to believe what parents tell them and to work in partnership with the family, and in the vast majority of cases this is the right approach. However, the safety of a child may well be dependent on the action of the practitioner, and so the action needed is to share a concern if one exists no matter how uncertain. In many ways this example is far too simplistic; the point of the exercise is that, in the vast majority of cases, rather than the incident itself being the deciding factor, the child's experience of childhood is significant - a significance which is best assessed from a number of perspectives.

Categories of abuse

The categories of abuse by which a child's name can be recorded on a child protection register are described in *Working Together*. Each section which follows will end with a brief case study intended to assist the reader in putting each category into a more realistic setting. While case studies are useful as a means of contextualising a theoretical discussion it is important to remember that the abuse of children can occur in an infinite variety of settings. The case studies are but one set of circumstances which should not be used as a list of indicators of when to be concerned.

Neglect

> The persistent or severe neglect of a child, or the failure to protect a child from exposure to any kind of danger, including cold or starvation, or extreme failure to carry out important aspects of care, resulting in the significant impairment of the child's health or development, including non-organic failure to thrive. (DoH 1991, p. 48)

This is often a difficult area for the practitioner as in some ways the conclusion that a child is being neglected comes as a result of concerns which develop over a period of time and results from the omission of parenting rather then from the commission of an abusive incident or series of incidents. The child may fail to meet developmental milestones for example: organic reasons are excluded, the parents are supported to improve their parenting skills, but still the care the child receives is neglectful. When to make the decision that this is a child protection concern and how much 'evidence' is needed to support that concern is a difficult one, as no incident may be present to act as a trigger. Some practitioners may be concerned that they will be seen as applying their own personal beliefs and standards of parenting and be reluctant to share concerns as a result.

Concerns that a child is or has been neglected can arise in many ways: a child with an illness for which appropriate and timely help has not been sought, lack of appropriate supervision which results in a child being injured, and insufficient nutrition which results in a child failing to thrive, for example, are neglectful acts in themselves with consequences to the child. It may help to keep in mind that ill-treatment in whatever form is sufficient reason to share a concern and that harm is harm however it is experienced by the child. It is the child's needs and developmental time-scale that remain the focus for decision making.

There have in recent years been a number of child deaths as a result of neglect, one of which is known as the case of Paul of Islington. Paul died in March 1993, following which his parents were convicted of manslaughter and cruelty, by neglect, of three other children. An inquiry, convened to look at the interagency involvement with Paul and his family, produced a number of findings significant to the lack of recognition of the significant harm being experienced by these children. Conclusions included the fact that key information was held by various agencies but not shared. When this information was collated into an interagency chronology of events the risk of significant harm was clearly demonstrated, underlining the need for interagency communication and the timely sharing of concerns.

The report produced as a result of the inquiry into Paul's death contains the following description:

> Photographs taken after his death show burns over most of his body derived from urine staining plus septicaemia, with septic lesions at the end of his fingers and toes. In addition he was suffering from pneumonia.
>
> It is impossible to imagine the level of suffering that this little boy experienced as death slowly occurred. (Bridge Child Care Consultancy 1995, p. 7)

It is a salutary fact that many practitioners had been involved with Paul's family over several years providing support of varying kinds. However, the lack of a child-centred view of the children's experience of parenting seems to have contributed to a lack of recognition of the harm they were suffering and the risks they faced.

Case study 1 - neglect

Jane, aged seven months, is the first child of Sally, a single mother aged 19 years. Darren, Jane's father is no longer living with Sally, having left the family home when Jane was two months old. Sally was the second of three children, all of whom were known to the social services throughout their childhood having spent varying amounts of time in local authority accommodation due to the inability of their parents to provide for their developmental needs as a result of chronic alcohol abuse.

Sally's pregnancy was uneventful resulting in the normal delivery of Jane at 39 weeks' gestation. At this time, Sally and Darren were living in local authority accommodation which the midwife and health visitor had visited reporting no concerns. Sally and Jane were discharged to the care of the midwife on the fifth day post delivery. Jane was bottle feeding.

At the point of handover from the midwife to the health visitor, the midwife commented that Sally was finding Jane demanding and difficult to cope with. She added that Darren took little part in the care of his daughter. The health visitor visited Sally and Jane weekly, discussing the need to feed Jane on demand and general issues of hygiene. Sally found the health visitor's visits intrusive, seeing her as interfering. Jane's weight dropped initially but slowly returned to the appropriate centile by the sixth week. Her six-week developmental assessment was satisfactory, although she was suffering from extensive nappy rash.

The health visitor advised Sally to attend the well-baby clinic every week to have Jane's weight checked. Her attendance was periodic and had ceased by the time Jane was three months old. As Jane's weight gain had been poor the health visitor made arrangements to visit the family at home when Sally told her that Darren had left.

Jane's weight gain continued to be poor which the health visitor discussed with Sally who reported that Jane was difficult to feed, often vomiting. She added that she had introduced baby rice to Jane's diet. The health visitor, concerned at Jane's poor weight gain and general lethargy, arranged for a GP's appointment that Sally did not keep. The health visitor made a follow-up home visit a number of times, however Sally was apparently not in. The health visitor discussed her concerns with the GP who reported that she had seen Sally recently complaining of being unable to sleep. Jane was by now four months old and had not attended for her routine immunisations.

The health visitor continued to attempt to visit Sally and Jane at home, eventually finding Sally returning from visiting her neighbour. Jane had been left alone in the flat during this time with a bottle propped against a pillow so she could feed. The health visitor advised Sally of the risk of Jane choking and said that on no account should Jane be left alone. The health visitor weighed Jane and found that her weight had dropped significantly in proportion to her birth weight and advised Sally to bring her to the GP's clinic that afternoon. Sally did not attend.

The health visitor discussed her concern with the GP and agreed to make a further home visit which she did the following day. Sally informed the health visitor that she was sick of her interfering, sick of being told that she couldn't care for her own baby and that she had just about had enough of Jane this and Jane that. She continued that she would not allow either the health visitor or the GP to see Jane any more. The health visitor continued to attempt to discuss the need to monitor Jane's weight but Sally was adamant.

The health visitor discussed her concerns with both the GP and her manager who agreed that if Jane could not be seen in the next week the health visitor would write to Sally informing her that she would be contacting the social services.

The day after Sally had told the health visitor that she no longer wanted Jane weighed, Sally and Jane arrived at the local A&E department. Jane had scalds to her face, back and arm which, Sally said, had been caused by a cup of tea. The triage nurse was concerned at Jane's appearance, commenting to the casualty officer that she was inappropriately dressed in a summer dress in January and was generally 'grubby'. On examination the casualty officer found extensive scalding to Jane's face, arm and back, extensive nappy rash and that she appeared pale, underweight and lethargic.

He discussed his concerns with Sally, suggesting that his colleague examine Jane. Sally agreed. He discussed Jane with the senior house officer (SHO), who examined her and suggested that she be admitted and seen by a paediatrician. Sally agreed and Jane was admitted. The paediatrician found Jane to be significantly underweight and that the scalds to her face, back and arm were more than the few hours old as Sally had reported and he became concerned at the general level of apparent neglect from which Jane seemed to be suffering. He discussed these concerns with Sally who became angry, saying that she was taking Jane home. The paediatrician advised Sally to allow Jane to stay in hospital so that tests could be made, but Sally refused. He continued that if she insisted on removing Jane he would have to contact the social services and suggested that it would be helpful if one of the hospital social workers came to see her on the ward so that between the three of them they could decide what to do for the best. Sally reluctantly agreed.

Sally saw the paediatrician and the social worker the following day and they discussed Jane's health, her weight, the way Sally had been feeding her and how she had come to be scalded. The social worker suggested said she would talk to Sally's GP and health visitor; the paediatrician said that Jane should stay in hospital until her weight improved and the results of the tests he had ordered were known. Sally refused to allow Jane to remain in hospital. The social worker and paediatrician advised against Sally taking Jane home and Sally said Jane could stay but that she wasn't having the health visitor or the GP involved and neither did she want the social services around. In discussion with the paediatrician, the health visitor and her manager, the social worker decided that a child protection conference was needed. The social worker discussed this with Sally who said they could do what they like but she wasn't having the health visitor or social worker telling her how to bring up her own kid.

The conference took place in the hospital seven days later, during which time Jane's tests had returned as within normal limits and her weight had improved significantly. The health staff invited to attend were the paediatrician, the triage nurse, Jane's nurse from the ward, the designated nurse for child protection and the health visitor. Sally was also invited to attend and, with some persuading, she agreed.

During the course of the discussion about Jane's needs Sally continued to deny that Jane had any problems with her weight and stated
that she would not allow the health visitor or social worker to visit
her at home.

It was decided that Jane's name should be recorded on the CPR
as she had suffered from significant harm, the cause of which was
neglect.

Commentary

Cases of neglect are often difficult to grapple with as concerns
develop over a period of time, the true extent of which may not be
evident until, or unless, an overall chronology of the case is
compiled.

In this case study there are many factors which suggest that Sally
may be a vulnerable parent and Jane a vulnerable child. It may help
to identify some of those factors in the following way.

Jane
- poor weight gain
- described by Sally as a difficult child
- feeding problems
- poor clinic attendance
- poor immunisation uptake
- has not attended GP appointments and developmental assessments
- left alone

Sally
- single, unsupported parent
- a recent separation from partner
- previously accommodated by local authority as a child
- resistant to advice
- unable to see Jane's needs above those of her own

In addition, the general situation of a family has a number of factors
which should alert the practitioner to the presence of additional
stresses. As above, it may help to identify some of these factors:

- delay and avoidance in seeking appropriate advice
- gradual withdrawal
- denial of access to practitioners

It is worth noting the cumulative effect of the identified factors and the escalating nature of concerns existing within this case study.

It is vital in cases such as these that the focus remains on the child and the child's experiences of childhood; Jane's experience is seen not only from her point of view at the time, but also the likely effects if the experiences are allowed to continue.

Note the effective level of communication between all practitioners involved and the prompt sharing of information and appropriate action taken. The reasons for convening a conference and the recording of Jane's name is Sally's refusal to work with practitioners, thus making it impossible accurately to assess the level of risk facing Jane and to address the underlying causes of her neglect.

Physical abuse

> Actual or likely physical injury to a child, or failure to prevent physical injury (or suffering) to a child including deliberate poisoning, suffocation and Munchausen's syndrome by proxy. (DoH 1991, p. 48)

Various research studies have shown that the highest risk of physical abuse to a child is in the first five years of the child's life and is most likely to be inflicted by the parents. The risk is largely equal for male and female children. The younger the child the more physically vulnerable, dependent and in some ways demanding he is. For example, a newborn child may need to be fed on a two-hourly basis, day and night, depriving the parents of valuable and much-needed sleep. As they grow older, children tend to test and explore, not only in terms of their environment - which can put them at risk of injury if not protected from their lack of awareness of danger - but also in terms of themselves, their psychological development and their interaction with others. It can perhaps be said that in the first five years of life a child is designed to test, explore and interact - to be, in varying degrees, the centre of attention with the demand for attention often immediate and insistent.

When other factors, such as poor housing, very young parents, a single parent, little family support and unemployment, are added to this scenario the effect, in short, can cause the child's parents to experience increasing degrees of stress, frustration and anger. This can undermine their ability to see the child's behaviour as developmentally appropriate, instead seeing the child as unreasonable, demanding and intentionally 'naughty'.

If parents have limited parenting skills, perhaps as a result of a poor parenting experience themselves, their own ability to withstand these frustrations can be compromised with the risk of a physical response, which is harmful to the child. Should a physical response result as a consequence of a loss of temper, frustration or exhaustion on the part of the parent then, generally speaking, the younger the child the more at risk he is of significant harm.

There are many dimensions to the discussion of what risks a child may face when experiencing a childhood in which violence is present which are beyond the remit of this book. Domestic violence can be especially significant and this will be expanded upon in the Conclusion, but a child will face many risks, mostly accidental, during his or her young life and it is important that practitioners remember this when considering child protection as a possibility. In addition, a child may sustain an injury inflicted by a parent which, when the context of the child's overall care is taken into account, is not considered to constitute significant harm. As identified in the Department of Health publication *Child Protection: Messages from Research* (DoH 1995b) it is not the incident that puts a child at risk of significant harm in the child protection sense, but the context in which that incident occurred. In general, children are at greater risk in a family characterised by high criticism and low warmth than a child whose family circumstance is one of high warmth and low criticism. This is true for all forms of abuse. However, the practitioner in the hospital setting may not be aware of the realities of a child's family circumstance and should keep child protection in mind, balancing the child's developmental ability and likelihood of sustaining an injury as presented in the way it is presented. It is also worth keeping in mind that, generally speaking, any fracture in a child under one year should be viewed with caution as they are developmentally unlikely to be involved in activities where such an injury is caused accidentally, unless involved in a road traffic accident.

In addition are injuries which may be caused by a loss of control by the parent: a child can be injured as a result of physical chastisement, for example. The issues of the appropriate use of physical punishment to correct a child's behaviour are beyond the remit of this book, suffice it to say that whatever the cause or explanation, harm is harm. If the practitioner is concerned that a child has been injured in this way he or she should discuss any concerns with the designated doctor or nurse.

Contained within the definition above is 'Munchausen's syndrome by proxy'. This is a psychological/psychiatric condition of the parent and is sometimes referred to as 'fictitious disorder'. Briefly, this is a situation in which the parent receives attention by using the child. This desire for attention can manifest itself in many ways. The parents may report symptoms they say they have observed, they may add foreign matter to the child's waste products, for example adding their own blood to the child's urine, or they may cause a child to 'have symptoms' by inducing an apnoeic attack or poisoning the child, for example. This is often a very difficult area for health practitioners as in order to 'diagnose' an illness in a child they listen to and believe what the parents are telling them. They must often exclude a variety of possible conditions as they investigate the cause. This process provides the parent with the attention he or she is seeking and subjects the 'well child' to unnecessary investigations. There is, of course, the fact that a child in this situation is just as likely to experience the usual childhood illnesses as any other child. How to differentiate between the child whose parents are genuinely presenting their child as ill in some way and the parent who is using the child to fill his or her own needs is extremely difficult. Added to this difficulty is the fact of the conclusion that a parent is suffering from this psychological/psychiatric condition developing as a result of the investigation undertaken on the child. The practitioner is advised to keep in mind that to protect a child in this circumstance, a circumstance in which there may be a significant risk of psychological harm, physical harm, induced disability and, on occasion, death of the child, they must 'think the unthinkable'.

Case study 2 - physical abuse

Casey, aged three months, is the second child of Janet, a primary school teacher, and Robert, a computer programmer. Casey's sibling is Josh, aged three years. The family live in an owner-occupied, three-bedroom, semi-detached house not far from the local general hospital.

Casey arrived at the A&E department as a result of a GP referral. His mother had taken him to the well-baby clinic for a routine weight check when the health visitor became concerned at the lack of movement in his left leg and the discomfort he was in when his leg was touched or moved in any way. She asked Janet if she had noticed this but Janet showed surprise, saying she didn't know what the matter could be. She agreed to see the GP who felt that an X-ray would be necessary and advised her to take Casey to the local A&E department.

On arrival Janet was concerned about Casey and anxious that she hadn't noticed anything wrong. She explained to the nurse that

Josh was very jealous of his new little brother and could be rough with him. The casualty officer examined Casey and referred him for X-ray that revealed a spiral fracture of his left femur. The casualty officer discussed this with the SHO who expressed concern that this was a non-accidental injury (NAI). A paediatrician was called and asked for an opinion.

The paediatrician confirmed that this could be an NAI and agreed to see Casey and his mother in A&E. Meanwhile, the nurse who had stayed with Janet and Casey at Janet's request talked to Janet about how her new baby and Josh were getting along. Janet explained that she was worried by Josh's reaction to Casey and wondered if it had anything to do with him recently starting at nursery and Janet returning to part-time work. The paediatrician then arrived and told Janet of Casey's fracture. Janet was distressed and said that it must have happened when she was changing him or perhaps Josh had hurt him when she was not looking. The paediatrician continued that sometimes babies can have a problem which means that their bones fracture very easily, but that it was unusual. He continued that this kind of injury was more usually caused by a pulling and twisting movement needing more force, such as that would be used when changing a nappy or when dressing a child. He also continued that it was unlikely that a three-year-old child would have done this. Janet became tearful and said that this was all she needed with the new house, going back to work, Josh having temper tantrums every five minutes and Robert working all the overtime he could get. The paediatrician said that he wanted Casey to be admitted so that his fracture could be sorted out and to have some tests done. He continued that he would have to talk to the social services because this was the kind of injury that could have happened when parents are under a great deal of stress and to see if there was any help that could be offered to the family. Janet agreed, and Casey was admitted. The paediatrician spoke to the social services and it was agreed that he and a social worker would see Janet and Robert as soon as possible.

Two hours later Robert arrived on the ward and spoke to Janet, who explained what the paediatrician had said. Robert became angry, demanding to know from the nursing staff exactly what was going on and what right the paediatrician thought he had to say that he or his wife abused their kids. He continued that he was taking his wife and son home and that there was nothing anyone could do about it. The nurse to whom Robert had said this tried to talk to him about Casey's need to stay and said that she would try to get hold of the paediatrician who could explain. Robert agreed to wait but said that it had better not be long. Janet by this time was crying and the nurse allocated to Casey stayed with her. The paediatrician arrived and saw Janet and Robert in the ward office. He explained to Robert all that he had said to Janet, adding that he had spoken to the social services and arranged to see both Robert and Janet the next day with a social worker at a time that would suit both of them. He continued that in the meantime it was best for Casey to stay in hospital and that Janet could stay with him. Robert, although very angry at this point, agreed and arranged to return the following day. Janet stayed with Casey.

Whilst on the ward Janet told Casey's nurse that she and Robert had not been getting along and that she was trying to keep everything together. She had no idea how this could have happened to Casey and said that it must have been Josh.

The following day the paediatrician and a social worker saw Robert and Janet as arranged. They talked about Casey and how his injury could have happened - both Robert and Janet said it must have been Josh. Robert continued that they did not need any help from the social services and would be taking Casey home as soon as he was well enough. The social worker explained that as Casey's injury was unlikely to have happened accidentally and because there was no real explanation, a child protection conference had been arranged and that both Robert and Janet would be invited to attend.

Robert, although angry, agreed to allow Casey to remain on the ward and agreed to attend the conference with his solicitor. The conference recorded Casey's name on the CPR under the category of physical abuse. Health staff invited to attend were the paediatrician, the nurse who first saw Casey in A&E and the ward nurse, together with the designated nurse for child protection.

Commentary

In cases where there is a clear injury such as that sustained by Casey, with a positive diagnosis of NAI, it is of vital importance that health practitioners convey that diagnosis in a prompt, clear and unequivocal manner to social services. The addition of an explanation may also be helpful as in such cases the social services will be dependent upon the nursing and medical practitioners to assist them on their most appropriate course of action. It is important to note that social services will make their own assessment, however that can be greatly informed by the diagnosis of the healthcare practitioner.

In this case study Casey has already sustained a significant injury, the cause of which is unresolved. It is reasonable to believe that Casey may be of further risk as a result of the parent's denial of the diagnosed cause of his fracture. Without their acknowledgement, even in part, it can be very difficult for practitioners to work with a family in order to address the factors which may have led to Casey being injured in this way, thus preventing, or at least minimising, the recurrence of a similar event.

When faced with articulate, seemingly caring and distressed parents it is all to easy for the practitioner to lose sight of the child's needs and focus solely on support for the parents. Whilst working in partnership with parents is to be encouraged, the primary focus must be the welfare of the child.

Sexual abuse

> Actual or likely sexual exploitation of a child or adolescent. The child may be dependent and/or developmentally immature. (DoH 1991, p. 49)

A child of either sex can be sexually abused at any age. That abuse can consist of many forms of behaviour from inappropriate touching, exposure to sexual activity or pornographic material, external genital contact and masturbating an adult to penetration. That penetration can be digital, with the use of foreign objects or with a penis, and can be oral, anal or vaginal. The perpetrators of sexual abuse can be male or female, of any age and it is most likely that the offender will either be a member of the family or known to it, such as a babysitter or youth leader. Intrafamilial abuse - abuse within one family that extends through generations - can exist and may extend from an abusive patriarch such as a grandfather. Although this will be 'organised' it should be seen as different from paedophile rings and similarly organised sexual abuse

Organised sexual abuse is comparatively rare, although it does occur and can be extremely sophisticated, involving many adults and children. Practitioners should remember that sexual abuse includes the use of a child or young person in prostitution. Ritualistic abuse or satanic abuse also exists, but the use of ritualistic or satanic beliefs, paraphernalia and behaviours is more likely to be to disguise, justify and reinforce the abuse rather than originating the abuse. All sexual abuse may have an element of ritual, as may any behaviour, and this is used to control the victim.

The range of abuse that can be considered within this category is considerable and is rarely 'diagnosed' by the presence of physical symptoms alone. In assessing the risk to a child or young person those who specialise in child protection take into account very many psycho/social issues and the consequences to the child or young person of action they may take. In the main, the hospital-based practitioner is unlikely to be presented with a child or young person whose symptoms leave them in no doubt that sexual abuse has occurred. Exceptions to this may be a child or young person whose physical condition is suggestive of forced penetration, for example a young child with anal and or vaginal tearing, the presence of seminal fluid, or, occasionally, a child or young person who discloses - although this is unusual. Should the practitioner be concerned that a child or young person may have been abused in this way he or she should not attempt to examine the child or young person unless specially trained to do. There may be exceptions to this such as the need to undertake procedures to maintain the child or young person's health and/or minimise further damage - advice should be taken from the designated doctor or nurse.

Case study 3 - sexual abuse

Mary's father, Graham, a police officer, first started touching her in a way she didn't like when she was six years old while her mother, Claire, a nurse, was in hospital having another baby, Kevin. This touching started as play fighting when Graham would tickle her under her clothes and sometimes touch her in between her legs. She 'sort of liked this', but wasn't sure. Gradually this play fighting developed with Graham encouraging Mary to tickle him in his trouser pockets saying that if she found any money she could keep it. This was a special game that she and her daddy played, mostly when he put her to bed. Over a period of two years this play fighting developed to Graham stroking Mary's tummy and thigh and then to putting his finger inside Mary's vagina. Like before, she 'sort of liked' this, but again wasn't sure. Graham constantly reassured her that it was okay and what Daddies did when they loved their daughters in an extra-special way.

When Mary was ten years old Graham attempted to penetrate her vagina with his penis. This caused Mary a great deal of pain and frightened her considerably. As before, Graham reassured her that this was okay and that next time she would like it. He tried again, succeeding this time, but still frightening Mary and causing her pain.

Mary was confused, frightened and lonely, feeling that although she loved her daddy and wanted to do what he liked, she did not like this new game. She could not tell her mummy because her daddy had said not to. Mary became a sad little girl, her performance at school began to suffer as she could not concentrate and she felt unable to talk to her friends any more so they stopped talking to her. Her mother couldn't understand why she was behaving this way, saying that she must stop being so naughty.

When Mary was 13 she took as many of her mother's sleeping pills as she could find and hid in the garden shed. She was brought in to A&E by ambulance having been found unconscious by Kevin. She had her stomach pumped out and was admitted.

The following day when the nurse was talking to her about her home and school and what she liked doing Mary began to cry, saying she didn't like Dad's games any more and that she wanted to sleep for ever so she wouldn't know when her dad wanted to play. The nurse asked her what she meant but Mary would say no more. The nurse reported this to the sister in charge who informed the designated nurse in child protection and the paediatrician. In discussion they agreed to inform the social services.

A social worker and female police officer went to see Mary on the ward and briefly confirmed the information, but did not go into too much detail. In discussion with the appropriate line managers it was agreed that Mary should be jointly interviewed, for which Mary's mother gave her permission. That afternoon Mary was taken to the local victim examination suite and, with her mother present, was interviewed by the social worker and police officer. Although nervous at first, Mary slowly began to relax and eventually gave a clear and precise disclosure which was recorded on videotape. Based on the nature of the disclosure Mary and her mother agreed to a medical examination that was undertaken by the police surgeon at the suite.

Later that same day Mary's father was arrested and interviewed. He denied the allegations. However, the arresting officers were satisfied they had enough information from the interview and medical examination to charge him. They released him on police bail not to return to the family home. Social services had made it clear that he should not return there, and he went to stay with relatives. Mary's mother had also made it clear that she did not want her husband home. She completely accepted what Mary had said and, although in shock, was able to manage the situation and protect Mary from contact with her father in the immediate future.

As Mary and her mother were willing to work with social services and Graham had been charged and was not allowed to return home, it was decided not to conference. Six months later Graham appeared at the Crown Court, pleaded guilty to indecent assault and was sentenced to six months' imprisonment.

Commentary

Cases of sexual abuse are often described by practitioners as causing them the most concern. For many, the difficulties of thinking the unthinkable once realised can be replaced with anger and disbelief that a child should have been abused in this way over a period of time - feelings that are in many ways entirely natural. In this case study, issues that may add to these feelings are that not only is it Mary's father who has systematically planned to abuse and who has carried out his plans as Mary has gradually become older and increasingly disempowered due to the effects of his grooming of her, but also by the fact that he is a police officer, a position of authority and trust. Important issues to note in this case study are the ways in which the practitioners were open to what Mary had to say, the way they took what she said seriously and acted in a prompt and supportive manner.

When assessing the level of risk Mary was facing the responsible manager took into account the protective and appropriate behaviour of Mary's mother and the removal of Mary's father from the home.

Emotional abuse

Actual or likely severe adverse effects on the emotional and behavioural development of a child caused by persistent or severe emotional ill treatment or rejection. (DoH 1991, p. 49)

Much has been written on this form of abuse. Some authors differentiate between emotional and psychological abuse (O'Hagen 1992), whilst others make less of the difference (Iwaniec 1995). The definition of abuse above makes no distinction between the two, talking in terms of emotional and behavioural development. Unless interested, hospital-based practitioners need not concern themselves with these complex discussions, however, a brief discussion of this potentially highly damaging form of abuse is useful in terms of understanding and recognition.

In brief, this form of abuse is concerned with the potential and actual damage caused to essential mental faculties and processes such as memory perception, moral sense, attention, cognition and intelligence. These processes allow us to understand the world around us, how individuals fit into that world and informs and directs the way individuals interact. These processes are connected to individuals' senses of themselves and how people think of and value themselves, which in turn affects the way they react to the world around them and the way they are reacted to. In short, emotional and psychological development is the development of who a person is and the way they think and behave.

A child's emotional and psychological development is linked to the emotional and psychological environment in which they are raised. The parents of a child whose responses to that child are emotionally inappropriate and inconsistent over a sustained period of time, particularly in the early years of the child's life, are likely to create an environment of inconsistency, unpredictability and confusion for that child. This environment puts the child at risk of experiencing pervasive and nebulous fear and confusion, undermining their ability to develop self-confidence and trust in themselves and others, and adversely affects their general wellbeing, ability to access education, and ability to socialise appropriately. As the above definition identifies, all forms of abuse have an emotional aspect to them; this category is used when it is the main or sole form of abuse.

Parents of such children will have distorted perceptions of their child and the realities of childhood. They may believe that it is the child who does not wish to be touched, cuddled and played with. In some families, it may only be one of a number of children who will be abused in this way. Indeed, the other children may come to echo this abuse in their behaviour and treatment of that child.

Hospital-based practitioners may have concerns that a child is being emotionally abused in many situations. They may observe inappropriate behaviour on the part of the parent. The child's behaviour may be a cause of concern. The nature of the interaction between parent and child may seem inappropriate. As before, whatever the concern and however unsure, the safest course of action for the child is to take advice and to share the concern.

Case study 4 - emotional abuse

Steven, aged four years and the only child of Pam and Brian, had always been described as a difficult and intentionally naughty boy by both his parents. He had been a difficult baby to feed, did not settle to a regular sleeping pattern and is still using nappies both day and night. The health visitor has monitored this family closely as she has been concerned at the way neither Pam or Brian seem to understand Steven's developmental needs for love, affection and time to be a child playing and learning about his environment.

Pam, a lecturer in mathematics at the local university, and Brian, a barrister, say that Steven has a good brain on his shoulders and needs to be taught how to learn in the most effective way and not to waste his time playing with no purpose.

In addition to her concerns relating to Steven's need to 'be a child', the health visitor has referred him to the speech clinic for generalised delay and the GP due to his poor growth. Steven attends the speech clinic with his mother on a regular basis, but in spite of encouragement from the speech therapist and the health visitor his mother has refused to allow him to attend a playgroup. Her reasons are that he can get all the stimulation he needs from adult company and being with other children will only encourage him to 'pick up bad and babyish habits'. Following the health visitor's referral to the GP Steven has been referred to the growth clinic at the local hospital.

Steven was brought to the A&E department by his father with a history of being unwell for around three days, hot, sleepy and not wanting his food. His father said that at first he and his wife thought it was nothing and didn't like to call or bother the GP for just one of those silly, childish things which are best left to work their way out of the system. The reason Brian gave for bringing Steven at this time was that the family were attending a wedding the following day and they wanted Steven to be well enough for them to attend as arranged. The triage nurse noticed that Steven was clearly pyrexial, lethargic and withdrawn. He sat in the chair next to his father looking down at his feet; neither Brain nor Steven seemed to communicate with each other. She commented on this to the casualty officer. On examination Steven was found to have a deep-seated chest infection which required his admission. Brian irritably agreed and said that he and his wife would return the following evening when they returned from the wedding.

Steven showed little sign of distress at his father's leaving and made little response when taken to the paediatric ward. The nurse allocated to Steven commented to the ward sister and the paediatrician that he seemed such a sad little boy, but that it might be because of the chest infection. Steven's medical condition had improved slightly by the following day, but he remained quiet and placidly compliant. The parents visited for one hour that evening, during which time they talked mostly to each other, Steven's nurse was surprised at how little they cuddled or touched the child. Steven himself made no move towards them, lying quietly in bed.

The following day Steven's medical condition had improved significantly, but still his nurse found him quiet, undemanding and highly reluctant to be with other children. The paediatrician had also commented on Steven's demeanour, his small stature and delayed speech. That afternoon Steven's mother visited the ward, spoke to the nursing staff, gave some books for her son and left, seeing Steven only briefly. The nurse noticed that the books she had left had a recommended reading age of seven.

The following day Steven was well enough to be discharged. His parents were called at home and a message left on their answering machine. At lunchtime a second call was made, and a third at around four o'clock. Steven's father phoned the ward at about five that evening saying that he and his wife would collect Steven the following day. In spite of encouragement to collect him that evening and an explanation that the best place for children is with their parents at home Brian insisted that it was not possible, saying that he and his wife would collect Steven tomorrow evening at seven.

In discussion with the ward staff the paediatrician decided to take advice from the social services as to his concerns at the emotional care Steven was receiving. He did this by telephone and an arrangement was made for a social worker to talk to Steven's parents with the paediatrician when they came to collect him. In the meantime the social worker would contact the health visitor.

The following morning the social worker rang the health visitor and explained her concerns. The social worker and the paediatrician met with Steven's parents that evening. Pam and Brian were surprised at their concerns, feeling that they were unfounded as they knew their son. They left with Steven.

The following day the health visitor visited the family by arrangement, and again talked to Steven's parents of his need to be with children of his own age and for developmentally appropriate treatment. Neither Brain nor Pam felt that she was being realistic and said that Steven would need to learn the value of hard work and independence from an early age if he were to succeed. They continued that it was for them to ensure that this happened.

The health visitor discussed her concerns with her manager and they decided to contact the social services as the health visitor felt that Steven was experiencing emotional abuse. The health visitor arranged to visit the family with a social worker. Both Pam and Brian repeated the comments they had made the previous day, continuing that they no longer needed the services of the health visitor or the social worker.

In discussion with the health visitor, her manager and the social worker's manager it was decided to convene an initial conference. Health staff were invited to attend, as was the health visitor, paediatrician and Steven's nurse from the ward.

Commentary

There are many factors identified in this case study which suggest that Steven may be at risk of emotional abuse. As with the first case study, it may be helpful to distinguish between the issues that relate to Steven and those that relate to his parents.

Steven's parents have described him as a difficult/naughty, boy taking personally what could be described as developmentally appropriate behaviour. This can in some cases lead to scapegoating, in that the parents hold the child responsible for issues which the child is developmentally unable to effect. Steven's parents are unable to see his developmental needs for love, affection and time to be a child, instead projecting on him their desires to have an academically successful child. This style of parenting risks Steven experiencing a sense of failure, lack of self-confidence and self-worth. In addition, his parents are unable to see his needs for peer-group socialisation. The needs of his parents during his illness to attend a social function took precedence over Steven's needs for his parents and the trauma he might experience from that separation.

Steven's behaviour includes a number of factors that rightly caused the health practitioners concerns, such as his poor speech development, his rather withdrawn, quiet and undemanding behaviour in hospital, his lack of interaction and his lack of distress at separation from his parents. Note also the way the practitioners liaise with each other, recording and sharing their observations of Steven's behaviour, the behaviour of his parents and the nature of their interaction.

Chapter 6
Collecting the evidence

Introduction

This chapter takes the practitioner through the referral and investigation stages, highlighting the shared responsibility of all those involved in the child protection process to collect appropriate evidence and feed it to those leading the investigation. This does not mean that hospital-based staff have a specific responsibility to collect evidence, but rather that there is a responsibility to be aware of the need to recognise and retain any information that may be essential to protecting a child and to share it. This chapter will not only highlight the importance of protecting information collected in hospital, but also discuss how other evidence is gathered during an investigation, the various forms this may take, and the uses to which it may be put. In Chapter 9 there will be a more specific examination of how this evidence may be used in both the civil and criminal court settings.

Traditionally, evidence may be seen as the significant information or material collected by the police with which the authorities gain a successful conviction in a court of law. The importance of clear, accurate, recorded evidence is as true in child protection investigations as in any other, but the evidence is not simply the substance of a successful action in the criminal or civil court, but also the basis upon which the child protection investigation and outcomes will be based. Gathering the evidence upon which decisions are made, at strategy meetings, case conferences, planning meetings and ultimately in court, is the responsibility of every practitioner involved with the child and family. It is essential that practitioners have a clear idea of what may be evidence, how it should be recorded, when it should be passed on, and to whom, and how it will be used.

The first step must always be to protect the child; while it is important to keep in mind that any evidence may be needed later, the child must be the first priority. It goes without saying that the practitioner must see to the child's immediate medical needs. If they have come into the A&E department, or have been admitted to the ward, then it is likely they will require medical care, possibly urgently. Once this is done there must be the opportunity to consider any concerns you may have gained during treatment or contact with the child and family. Child abuse may only be one possibility, but should perhaps be the last to be dismissed while concerns or uncertainties exist.

Referrals and recording

If there is any doubt that a child needs protection referral then informal discussions should take place between the hospital practitioner and social services. Often, while the referral is not seen as child protection it will give a chance for services to be mobilised and to provide a family in need with support which may prevent future problems. In general social services departments will be flexible - while retaining the need to keep the child's needs and safety as paramount, they will also recognise that there are several ways of responding to concerns which may facilitate the required outcome.

If a formal child protection referral is made then this should go to the appropriate social services department. This may be made to the nearest office, perhaps to a duty team, reception and assessment team, or child protection team. Many hospitals will have their own social work teams, and some authorities have emergency duty teams for weekends and out-of-hours referrals. It is important that the practitioner is aware of the local referral route. The receiving social worker will require as clear and as detailed a referral as possible based on the presenting concerns, any relevant history and the impressions gained by the medical staff involved. Impressions can be significant, but must be well founded. Do not hold things back because you are uncertain, but share your uncertainty. Specific medical evidence should be precise where possible. If there are still further tests or X-rays to be done then make it clear that the evidence is up to a particular point in time and say if there is a differential diagnosis. If you are making a telephone referral, if possible, confirm the information by fax as soon as you can.

It is vital that the practitioner records the information concerning the child in the medical or nursing record system appropriate to the hospital. Recording is an essential part of the child protection processes whichever agency you work for. It will be in the notes practitioners keep that much of the evidence for future reference will be contained. It is possible that the first involvement with a child will not be recognised for what it is, but that over months or even years a chronology will build that will lead to a referral after the child is readmitted for a similar injury. Therefore, even if the case is not clearly NAI the information should still be recorded for possible future reference. It is imperative that each piece of information is accurately recorded, making clear its source, the date and time when it was collected, and where appropriate quoting what was said.

The Access to Personal Files Act 1987 enables individuals to have access to manually kept information kept about them, while the Data Protection Act 1984 provides for computer-based information. Family members subject to an investigation may well want to see what is written about them and ask to have access to that information. It is therefore important that an agency has an appropriate system for dealing with such requests, and that the practitioner is mindful that those they are writing about could see the information. Most practitioners would argue that client/customer access to records is to be encouraged and, in fact, aids good practice. It should not discourage the practitioner from keeping accurate notes of their findings and conclusions, but rather encourage good practice in record keeping.

Telling the family that a referral has been made is good practice, but the practitioner making the referral may understandably find this difficult. While the impact on the future success of intervention of keeping the family informed and working with them in partnership cannot be underestimated, practitioners have to be aware of the need to protect the child and members of staff. Therefore, however desirable it may be it is not always wise or possible to tell parents that a child protection referral is being made. In certain cases, such as Munchausen's syndrome by proxy, or when there is immediate risk of further abuse actually taking place in the hospital, then the family should not be told. It may also impede the investigation if an alleged abuser has prior knowledge of the investigation. It is vitally important that the practitioner speaks to the designated nurse or doctor and, where appropriate in consultation with social services, makes the decision as to informing the parents of the referral. This decision, like all others, should then be recorded alongside the reasons for making it.

Child protection investigations

The social services department to which a formal child protection referral is made will have in place a system for receiving and recording the information and initiating the investigation. The first priority is to establish if the child is in immediate need of protection. If, for instance, a child has left the hospital to return home with his or her parents then it may be necessary to visit the home to ensure the child's safety. When there is enough concern to believe that the child may suffer significant harm if not removed from the home then social services may either persuade the parents to agree to the local authority accommodating the child or, if such agreement is unlikely, the social services may apply for an emergency protection order or enlist the assistance of the police for the child to be taken under police protection. Even if the child remains in the hospital it is important to make certain the child is safe and here again it may be necessary to take legal action to provide for the child's safety.

However, whenever possible the child and family will remain together and the investigation will be conducted in partnership with them. Inevitably, children and families who are suddenly the subject of a child protection investigation will be shocked, possibly angry and scared. An open approach, with procedures and actions being clearly explained, will assist in reducing suspicion and fear.

Once it has been established that the child is safe the investigating social worker will follow the departmental procedures and in particular begin gathering evidence from the other agencies that may know and have contact with the family. This may include schools, the GP, the health visitor, the NSPCC and further contact with the hospital-based staff. The police will also be contacted and after a strategy discussion a decision will be made as to whether or not it should be a joint or single agency investigation when it will be left to social services to pursue inquiries. Strategy discussions can vary from the simplest telephone exchange of views between responsible managers to a substantial interagency plan, depending on the nature and complexity of the alleged or suspected abuse. The hospital-based practitioner should be part of these discussions when the child remains in A&E or on the ward.

The pivotal information at this stage is likely to be that which is provided by the child either verbally or in the form of physical evidence. If appropriate the child will be spoken to initially either by a social worker and/or a police officer to explain what is happening and to determine the nature of the suspected or alleged abuse. It may then be decided to jointly interview the child under the *Memorandum of Good Practice* (Home Office/DoH 1992).

The child's evidence

The criminal law in particular has not always looked favourably on the child or given much credibility to what the child has to say. In the criminal system adults not only had power through the abuse they inflicted, but also in the way society and the law in particular dealt with allegations and treated the children making them. It was only in 1988 that the Criminal Justice Act took a significant step for children involved in criminal court proceedings by abolishing the assumption that a child was an 'incompetent' witness and by making it possible for children to give evidence through the use of television links. In the wake of this and the undoubted impact of the Act other non-legislative changes can be detected, in areas such as training, interagency cooperation and shared operational procedures.

In 1991 the Criminal Justice Act put an end to the right of the accused to cross-examine the child and allow a video-recorded interview to stand as evidence-in-chief. The Home Office and Department of Health jointly published the *Memorandum of Good Practice* in 1992 which gives professional guidance to those interviewing children to obtain evidence for court. The Memorandum is an extremely practical guide for police officers and social workers conducting interviews. It has been written with a clear child focus. The video-recorded interview should broadly equate with a written statement of events in which the child was a victim or a witness.

Video-recorded interviews with children may be admitted in a criminal trial under Section 32A of the Criminal Justice Act 1988 (as amended by the Criminal Justice Act 1991). Section 32A allows a video recording of an interview with a child witness of certain sexual or violent offences to be used in court, where it relates to any matter in issue in the proceedings, in trials at the Crown Court or youth court. The offences covered by Section 32A are as follows:

- any offence which includes assault on, or injury or a threat of injury to a person
- an offence under Section 1 of the Children and Young Persons Act 1933 (cruelty to a person under the age of 16)
- any offence under the Sexual Offences Act 1956, and the Indecency with Children Act 1967

- Section 54 of the Criminal Law Act 1977, or the Protection of Children Act 1978
- any offence which consists of attempting or conspiring to commit, or the aiding, abetting, counselling, procuring or inciting the commission of, an offence.

The video recording of the child's evidence recorded during the interview is only admissible where:

- the child is not the accused
- the child is available for cross-examination (assuming the proceedings get that far), and
- rules of court requiring disclosure of the circumstances in which the recording was made have been properly complied with.

There will be interagency discussions, normally between the police and social services, prior to an interview, and it should only take place when it is essential to a criminal investigation. The child, more often than not accompanied by a parent or appropriate adult, will normally be taken to the local victim examination suite (VES). The suites are especially designed in a way that should allow the child to relax and feel safe. The interview room should be like a sitting room, with toys and refreshments readily available and the cameras and microphones discreetly placed. The suite will also usually contain a medical examination room.

In practice it tends to be the police officer who will lead the interview, but the social worker may do so and, often, experienced practitioners will share the interview. Those workers involved have to always be aware that the videotape will be given in evidence and therefore they must concentrate on asking open questions without leading or encouraging the child. If the child is distressed or unreceptive it can be difficult to retain this objective approach, but it is important to remember that the court may reject the evidence if not obtained appropriately.

In Chapter 9 the child as a witness in the criminal court process is considered.

Medical evidence

The hospital-based practitioner has the opportunity to supply the investigation with essential information, but has to remember that the investigating social worker will not have specific medical knowledge and therefore information should be precise and understandable. Information that is confused or too complicated will hinder and possibly prevent an investigation from achieving a successful outcome. It may put the child at greater risk if, for instance, the information is ambiguous. As with a referral, any information given over the telephone should be confirmed by fax as soon as possible.

Other medical information may come from the police surgeon following the examination of the victim and from the family's GP. If the child is in hospital, then the police surgeon will often go there to conduct the examination. Alternatively, the child may be taken to the local victim examination suite, where the medical examination can take place, often in proximity to the joint interview.

While medical and forensic evidence can be essential, it is also important to be aware that abusers can be extremely devious and manipulative and attempt to disguise or tamper with evidence. This can be true in a case of Munchausen's syndrome by proxy and experienced sex offenders can become forensically aware through experience and are careful not to leave forensic evidence, for instance by wearing condoms during intercourse. They may learn much of their abuse craft from other offenders when serving a sentence in prison, or from reading about cases in books or through the media. Crime, especially serious often horrendous incidents, has become a popular diet for the inquisitive public, and fictional presentations on television, film and in books endeavour to become as realistic as possible. New techniques of investigation are given a great deal of exposure - DNA is an excellent example. This does not mean that they become quickly redundant, or that offenders in general become sophisticated, it means that practitioners have to be aware that the offender has a craft at which he works.

Other evidence

The police will use a variety of methods to gather evidence which may be of value to a criminal investigation and which may also be used to support the child protection investigation and, at a later date, civil legal action. For instance, photographic techniques, both still and video, will be used to record that unearthed by the forensic and medical experts. The child may be photographed, or the accommodation in which he or she lives. Photographic evidence can be used to great effect in both criminal and civil proceedings - bruises and injuries fade and cannot be brought to court, but photographs can. Photographic evidence can perform a unique part in bringing the

Photographic evidence can perform a unique part in bringing the scenes, often months or even years before, to life for the benefit of the court. In cases of neglect, photographs taken of the child's accommodation - such as a bare bedroom with urine-soaked bedding or an empty fridge - can be powerful, far more effective than the written or spoken word. It may be important not only to take photographs of the child's room, but also of the parents' accommodation if they lived in much better conditions - comparative photographs are extremely useful.

The police may wish to collect statements from any individual who may have witnessed a crime or have some specific knowledge of what has happened - another reason for practitioners to keep accurate notes of anything they may have seen or heard or believed to have happened.

Assessment

The investigating social worker will prepare an initial assessment based on the evidence they have been able to gather and setting out the level of risk and the actions that need to be taken to protect the child. The assessment should also contain a chronology, not only of the most recent events, but stretching back as far as is possible and appropriate in order to gain a broad picture. A pattern of abuse may then begin to appear that was not apparent with a single reported incident. The assessment may change as more becomes known about the family and how the family responds to the investigation. If there is to be a conference then the assessment will form the basis of the report presented there by the investigating social worker. It will also be the starting point should social services decide that court action is necessary (this will explored further in Chapter 9). Where possible the assessment will include the family members and, in particular, the wishes of the child. If there is not to be a conference then the information gathered may be used to assist in delivering services to the family.

A significant number of investigations will result in the suspicion or allegation being unsubstantiated, or not proven. During the investigation it may become apparent that there are no concerns, or that while there is some cause for concern it does not reach the threshold where a conference or agency involvement is necessary. There will also be cases in which there may be suspicions, but not enough evidence to take action. These will remain on file should further information come to light enabling social services to act.

Case study 5a

The following main study will be followed through Chapters 6, 7 and 8, taking the reader through the key elements of the child investigation process and its outcomes. The case study concerns a family in which domestic violence is the cause of the significant harm experienced by the children. Whilst it is fair to say that in some cases of domestic violence the violence is committed by a woman towards a man, these cases are rare. The vast majority of domestic violence is committed by men towards women and is the most common cause of serious injury and death of women as a result of violence.

Sharon, aged 23, has three children: Sophie, aged seven, Elizabeth, aged five, and Andrew, aged five days. Peter, aged twenty-nine, is the father of Andrew, while Sophie and Elizabeth have different fathers. Peter is a self-employed architect and local politician. The couple met at a fundraising event and soon became good friends. The friendship developed and Sharon found herself pregnant with Andrew. When Sharon told Peter of the pregnancy he suggested that they move in together and Sharon happily agreed. Sophie and Elizabeth did not take to Peter, finding him frightening, and they frequently refused to talk to him or to do as he asked. Sharon was a little concerned especially at the way Peter seemed to be intolerant of the girls, describing them as wilful and out of control. Sharon did not like Peter disciplining the girls, especially when he shouted at them. This had been a frequent cause of friction between the two of them, escalating at times to Peter accusing Sharon of being a bad mother, unable to control her children, and his insistence that the girls be taught how to behave, if not by Sharon then by him. On occasions Peter had smacked one or other of the girls and at one time had pushed Sharon out of the way when she attempted to intervene. This incident resulted in Sharon sustaining a bruise to her leg as she fell against a chair. On seeing the bruise the following morning Peter had expressed his sorrow, saying that it would not happen again if Sharon would only learn to control the girls.

When Sharon was eight months pregnant an argument began between Peter and the girls and Sharon attempted to pacify the situation. Peter became even angrier, saying that Sharon was too soft on the girls and should exercise more control. He also said that she should support him instead of undermining him. Sharon attempted to reason with Peter, who became angrier still. When Sharon attempted to leave the room Peter pulled her back, telling her never to turn her back on him, and pushed her into a chair. He then hit her across the face and abdomen. Sophie and Elizabeth, who were both present, were now crying and clinging to their mother. Sharon was crying but still attempting to leave the room with the two girls. Peter pulled Sharon out of the chair and shouted that she was to do something with those screaming brats or he would. Sharon managed to take the girls into their bedroom where they eventually settled. The girls and Sharon slept together that night, while Peter slept in his and Sharon's room. The following morning Sharon was woken by an intermittent pain in the lower part of her back, and she also had bruising to her left cheek and abdomen. The pains in her back became more painful and she called Peter. Peter came in, saw Sharon's face, broke down into tears and promised never to touch her again if she would forgive him. Sharon, by now in considerable discomfort, agreed. Peter took the girls to a friend who had agreed to look after them when Sharon went in to labour, then took Sharon to hospital.

Peter and Sharon arrived unannounced at the labour ward. The ward was busy and a flustered midwife showed them into a cubical. She checked Sharon's contraction rate, confirmed that the baby's head was engaged and said she would return shortly to do a vaginal examination. She asked if Sharon and Peter had brought Sharon's notes with her and Peter told her not to be so stupid - did she not think that they had better things to think about than bits of paper at a time like this. The midwife apologised, and Peter settled. The midwife returned, undertook an assessment and found that Sharon was in the early stages of labour. Sharon was transferred to a labour suite. When the midwife had settled Sharon and made her comfortable she asked Sharon how she got the bruises to her face and abdomen. Sharon looked at Peter and said she had fallen. The midwife recorded her observations in the records together with Sharon's explanation and Peter's earlier behaviour.

The midwife discussed how the couple wanted her to manage the labour. Both Sharon and Peter said that they wanted as natural a birth as possible - no drugs, Peter added, continuing that Sharon had had so many drugs with her last two labours that she had 'missed' the birth. The midwife asked Sharon if she also felt that way and Sharon, looking at Peter, agreed. The labour progressed with Sharon coping well until her contractions become so painful that she asked the midwife what sort of pain relief she could have. Peter immediately reminded her of the agreement that they had made, saying that he had promised her that if she lost her resolve during the labour that he would stop her giving in to what are, after all, only natural pains. Sharon agreed to continue without pain relief in spite of the midwife attempting to discuss the matter further, suggesting that gas and air might help and would not affect the baby.

Half an hour later Sharon's was finding it difficult to cope with the pains and again asked for pain relief. As before, Peter reminded her of the promise she had made and said that she could hurt the baby if she was weak and gave in. Sharon became tearful, saying that she could not cope with the pains any more. The midwife handed her the gas and air mask which Peter removed with some force, telling the midwife that she had no right to undermine him and that if she continued he would make an official complaint. The midwife responded by advising Peter that she had a duty to both Sharon and her unborn child and that Sharon needed pain relief now to allow her to rest for when she would have to start to push. Sharon asked again for pain relief, but Peter refused to release the mask. Despite encouragement from the midwife Peter continued to keep hold of the mask. The midwife called the doctor.

The doctor arrived and discussed the need for pain relief with Peter who readily agreed, saying that the midwife had blown his concern for Sharon out of all proportion. He then turned to Sharon and said that all she had to do was to say she needed help.

One hour later Sharon gave birth to a boy, whom she and Peter had decided to call Andrew. Soon afterwards mother and baby were transferred to the postnatal ward. After staying a further half an hour Peter left to collect the girls and return home.

Peter returned that evening to find Sharon breast-feeding Andrew. Sharon asked how the girls were and if they had settled okay, continuing that she had been worried at the way that they might still be upset. Peter said that they were fine and if they had been upset it was down to her for not raising them to respect their elders and betters and for not supporting him. Sharon apologised and asked him if he wanted to hold his son. She passed Andrew to Peter, but the baby quickly became restless. Sharon suggested that he might still be hungry and asked to have him back. Peter said that this was how the girls come to be so spoilt, by always getting what they wanted and he would not allow a son of his to grow up in the same way. Andrew began to cry and Sharon got up to take him out of Peter's arms, but he pushed Andrew at her. Sharon lost her balance and she and Andrew fell against the bed. The midwife who witnessed this came over, asking if all was well and suggesting that she look at Andrew, who was by now crying loudly. Peter reminded her that Andrew was his son and that he would decide if anyone needed to look at him. Sharon attempted to intervene but Peter told her to keep quiet and to stop undermining him. The midwife left to take advice. She spoke to the designated midwife who suggested that she contact the paediatrician, inform her of what had happened and ask her to examine Andrew as soon as possible, then to return to Sharon, Peter and Andrew and continue to encourage Peter to allow her to examine Andrew. She also reminded her to record all she had seen and said she would contact the hospital social work team.

Commentary

There are a number of key points demonstrated in the above which can be summarised as follows. The early part of the case study identified the presence of a level of friction caused by Peter's view of the girls' behaviour and his expectation that Sharon should correct this behaviour in order to avoid his irritation and anger. This can be seen as Peter holding Sharon and the girls responsible for his loss of control. In addition it has been shown that Peter is willing to use physical action in a situation of conflict involving Sharon and the girls.

Whilst in the labour ward it became apparent that Peter was prepared to allow Sharon to continue her labour in the absence of the pain relief requested by her and advised by the midwife. Both this example and the one above can be seen to demonstrate Peter's tendency to dominate.

The midwife carefully recorded all that she had observed in her notes. She later used these records to produce a report for the conference that included her name, qualifications and clinical experience, an account of and the reason for her involvement with Sharon, Peter and Andrew, the nature of that involvement - clarifying whether the information she was sharing had been observed by her or was reported to her - and both Andrew and Sharon's health. She concluded with the level of risk she felt Andrew had been exposed to. She signed and dated her report.

Chapter 7
The child protection conference

Introduction

The child protection conference (hereafter the conference) is pivotal to interagency cooperation in child protection. It is the forum in which practitioners share and coordinate information and concerns about the child and family, assess the severity of abuse and neglect and evaluate the degree of risk. Social services (and the NSPCC) have the statutory powers to convene a conference. This is likely to be done when an initial investigation, known as a Section 47 investigation, has confirmed or suspected abuse or neglect, or to review an earlier decision to place a child's name on the local CPR. The conference is not there to decide if a person is guilty, which is for the court to consider and rule upon should court action be taken, but rather to focus on the needs and risks to the child or children concerned. While the conference should not get drawn into issues of guilt, it is important that it has a clear understanding of who has responsibility to protect the child from harm and whether they are capable of doing so.

The conference does not take place in isolation from the child protection process and nor should it be seen as a rubber stamp to a decision already made by social services. It is an integral part of the process and the impact it may have on that process cannot be underestimated. It is not simply the decision that will have importance, but the way the conference is managed and the atmosphere in which it takes place. These factors, amongst others, will contribute to the perception of the meeting's relevance held not only by the agencies attending but also by the child and the family. Ultimately the conference has an essential power, an influence that can enhance the chances of developing a successful partnership with the family.

Working Together and local procedures set out guidelines as to why and when a conference is to be called. To be effective there has to be clarity of purpose and a clear decision-making process. The conference arena is governed by and expected to fulfil statutory obligations for the protection of children. Local procedures, in most places prepared by the ACPC, dictate how the conference will be managed and define the expected outcomes. Through the workings of the ACPC and interagency procedures and training, those attending the conference should have shared values, a clear purpose, clear understanding of current child protection issues and an explicit child focus.

While conferences throughout England and Wales follow broadly similar procedures there will be variations on the theme. The conference is very far from being an exact science. Conferences held within the jurisdiction of the same local authority may be different. The larger the authority, such as a shire county, the greater the possible differences. Large authorities may be divided into areas each with its own CPR and local procedures. While one can prepare the reader for the basics of what will happen during a conference it is not possible to predict the exact process of the meeting or the atmosphere in which it will take place. It is important to recognise and work with, not avoid, conflict or difference, but if these are not properly managed then the conference may lose its objectivity and become an arena for unhelpful, even counterproductive, argument.

Atmosphere can be as important as process and content. It has to be remembered by all those present that the conference is not an end in itself, it is part of the child protection process in which working with parents in order to keep children safe within families is the ultimate aim. Court proceedings may often be necessary but are not inevitable - it is a minority of cases that involve such proceedings, although the number is growing. Parents attending a case conference have an opportunity to see agencies working together at first hand and the impression they get from the experience can greatly influence how effective future intervention will be. Presenting a united view based on the needs of the child is vital, as is the need to balance criticism where possible with positive comment. The last thing that should happen is the parents leave the conference having witnessed a fragmented debate or feeling isolated and without hope. If the conference can deliver the right message in the right way then it can be an effective and locomotive force for positive change.

Types of conference

There are two types of conference:

- the initial child protection conference
- the child protection review.

An initial conference should be convened only after an investigation under Section 47 of the Act into an incident or suspicion of abuse. Not all children who are the subject of an investigation where significant harm is identified will be the subject at conferences. An assessment will be made in the light of the presenting or possible harm, historical information, the relative seriousness of the harm, the risk of future harm, the attitude of the family towards the child and their willingness to work with the agencies, and the ability of the parents to protect the child. If it is felt that the child is safe from future harm then a conference may not be called and either the family will be offered appropriate services, or the case may be closed by the social services.

If there is a decision to conference then this should be convened as promptly as possible after the referral is received. The priority at the beginning of the investigation will always be to make certain the child is safe - once this is done the investigating social worker can concentrate on undertaking the assessment and making the arrangements for the conference. Once the initial conference has been convened the only decision it has to make is whether or not to register the child. Ideally the conference will agree an outline protection plan and nominate a key worker who will be responsible for carrying out the plan in partnership with staff from the other agencies involved.

The review conference is there to review the arrangements for the protection of the child, for instance after a comprehensive assessment, and to make changes to the child protection plan where necessary by considering current risks and needs in the family and whether the plan continues to protect the child. It reviews interagency cooperation and considers if the child should remain on the register or be deregistered. The usual interval between reviews will be three months, but should be no longer than six. A request for a review conference may be made at any time, by any agency, based on changes in the child's or family's situation. Once the child protection plan has been agreed a group of practitioners will be identified as essential contributors to the services going into the family. The key worker, in cooperation with these practitioners, will organise case discussions and planning meetings between reviews, the frequency determined by the complexity of the case.

Before the conference

The success of a conference will depend on the quality of the preparatory work undertaken by all those attending, but in particular by the investigating social worker or team and by the chairperson. It is the social worker who is responsible for ensuring that everyone with a relevant contribution to make has been invited and that all available information is collated and recorded. A conference may arise from a family that is already known to social services or from a new allegation of abuse or neglect. It may be possible to prepare in detail for a conference, but equally an urgent conference may be necessary where there is less time to gather information. However, the amount of information is not necessarily important - it is the quality and the nature of the information that is vital.

As described in Chapters 4 and 6, the investigating social worker will have carried out checks on the child and family concerned with relevant agencies and this should act as a signal to those agencies that an investigation is in progress and a conference is possible. Once the decision to hold a conference has been made, usually after discussion between the investigating social worker, team manager and service manager, then invitations will be sent out to the family, regular attendees if there are any, and other practitioners who may know the family or be able to offer relevant knowledge or skills to the conference. The calling of the conference should not come as a surprise to the family and they should be informed in person by the investigating social worker. In the section below on 'Parents and the family' suggestions are made as to how people should be informed, encouraged and assisted in attending the conference. Information given should include details about the conference and the child's and parents' rights. All practitioners involved should take on the responsibility to assist the family with understanding the conference process.

The physical nature of the venue is important not only to ensure accessibility, but also to encourage a balance between a businesslike discussion and a relaxed atmosphere. If possible this should be a regular venue, although conferences may be convened elsewhere to facilitate attendance, such as in a children's home or hospital if the conference concerns a newborn baby or child remaining on a ward. A large conference is difficult to manage and the investigating social worker will discuss the invitation list with the chairperson to make sure only those with essential information are invited. If a practitioner does not get an invitation to a conference and yet believes they have something useful to contribute they should contact the investigating social worker to discuss the issue. Practitioners may be asked to submit written reports rather than actually attending in order to reduce the number of those present. Most important, a large conference can overwhelm the family and this will not help in developing the partnership between family and practitioners that is essential to effective child protection. In addition, the practitioners present may feel they have not had a fair opportunity to express their views and debate the issues, and physically a large conference can be uncomfortable.

Conference membership

In Chapter 3 the roles of the individual child protection agencies were briefly examined. The conference is the central mechanism by which these agencies may work in harmony to protect children. Those attending the conference will generally fall into three groups: those practitioners attending because of the particular family involved, the family members, and specially invited specialist workers or 'experts'. Membership will be drawn from social services, health, police, education, NSPCC and probation and other agencies with a relevant contribution to make. Conferences are also able to access specialist advice that may include a lawyer with childcare experience from the local authority's legal section, interpreters and, if legal proceedings have begun, the *guardian ad litem*.

A number of different health practitioners may attend because of their knowledge of the family or their involvement with the incident that has led to the conference. These might include:

- GPs, who should attend all conferences on children and families known to them as they will usually have invaluable information about the child and family, often covering many years of involvement
- hospital doctors and nursing staff, who are often the first to suspect or identify the victims of abuse or neglect. Hospital-based practitioners can advise the conference on the diagnosis and the behaviour and the impression left by the family in the hospital

- health visitors and midwives, who are able to offer detailed knowledge of the child and parents and will often play a significant part in the protection plan, monitoring a child's health and development, often, in the case of the health visitor, for many years
- community psychiatric nurses, who may know a parent because of illness, or alcohol and drug misuse
- a member of the child and family therapy team or child psychiatric team, who may be invited either because they know the family or can offer particular input.
- a paediatrician or psychiatrist, for example, who can provide expert medical advice which has been requested either on the child or family members.

Health practitioners attending must focus on the needs of the child during the conference and give views based not only on their own experience, but also on the needs and wishes of the child and the need to protect that child from future harm.

As for social services, the investigating social worker will attend and possibly other relevant social services staff, either those already involved with the family or those likely to become involved. These may include family centre workers, specialists in working with children with disabilities and those experienced in the area of alcohol or drugs misuse.

As far as the broad spectrum of education is concerned, headteachers, teachers, special needs workers, nursery and playgroup workers and childminders will often know the child well and are well placed to observe evidence of abuse. Indeed, school-age children will often disclose to a close friend or teacher. Education welfare officers (education social workers) are able to provide information about the family, or both, especially the child's school attendance. However, teachers are only available during term time and education welfare officers have no access to school records during holidays, which can mean that a conference will lack important information about a child's educational progress.

The police will attend if they have initiated an investigation with the decision to take police protection or through liaison with the local social services department. Most police areas will keep social services informed of concerns about children and young people they come across during routine police work. They also will provide information on offenders living in the home or associated with the abuse.

It is also likely officers will attend the conference, having been co-workers with social workers in the initial investigation, and will report on the current state of the inquiry.

The probation service will rarely attend conferences unless directly involved with a member of the family, usually an offender either under supervision in the community or in prison. This person may be an abuser or suspected of abuse and the probation service can offer an invaluable insight into offending behaviour.

During the process of the investigation organisations or agencies other than those with statutory responsibility may provide useful information about the family's circumstances and representatives from these may be invited to the conference, for instance the local authority housing department or housing association, the local women's refuge, or voluntary organisations that can provide services to children and families. NSPCC staff may be invited to attend, possibly because of current involvement with the family, but more likely as consultants when not directly involved in the case. They may provide comprehensive assessments to inform decision making or resources such as family centres and family therapy.

The chairperson

Recognition of the importance of the conference chairperson has greatly increased during recent years with the widespread introduction of specific training for the role, clearer guidelines as to whom should take the chair and, in some areas, the introduction of independent chairs. The chairperson at an initial conference will normally be a senior member of the social services management team without line management responsibility for the case, often a service manager, and with detailed knowledge of child protection. A growing trend is towards the use of independent chairpersons, specifically recruited from outside social services and employed to act as chairperson at all or most conferences in that area. Some authorities will employ a panel of people to share this task, or second individuals from another agency such as the NSPCC.

The chairperson is vital. He or she ensures the conference prioritises the child's interests, clarifies the meeting's purpose and the roles of the people present, and enables each to contribute appropriately. In particular the chairperson should make sure the family members present understand statements being made by practitioners and have their own chance to voice an opinion. The chairperson has a responsibility to promote openness, understanding and cooperation, focusing on the task and encouraging a decision-making process based on the evidence before the conference.

The chairperson will be aware of conflicts that may exist between practitioners and the need to manage the meeting where necessary. For instance, a practitioner may believe that he or she has a special relationship with the family, or particular insight into the needs of the child. This may result in them battling with, or bullying the conference in an attempt to achieve what they believe is best. This is most likely to happen when a practitioner is not a regular attendee and is therefore not attuned to the way the conference operates. They may feel excluded and therefore attempt to 'get their way' in an inappropriate manner. Equally, a strong social worker or member of the core group can cajole or bully a conference towards their chosen conclusion.

When possible the same person should chair all case conferences concerning particular children and families, but because of pressure of work, leave and sickness this is often logistically impossible. Review conferences, for instance, might be chaired if not by an independent then by a social services team manager, but again without line management responsibility for the case. The chairperson and investigating social worker should have met prior to the conference so that they are both fully aware of the facts behind the case, difficulties that may arise during the conference and have some idea of the possible outcomes.

The minute taker

Adequate recording of discussions, facts, decisions, recommendations, tasks and interagency plans is essential, and for these reasons the task of minute taker is also vitally important. The minute taker performs a task that is often not fully appreciated by those other practitioners attending the conference. They will normally be an experienced member of social services administrative staff, trained specifically to be able to take minutes in an often difficult situation where accurate recording is essential. Traditionally minutes have been taken in shorthand, but more recently mobile computers have been used in order to facilitate faster recording. This also saves time when it comes to preparing the finished minutes.

The minute taker will usually be responsible for the provision of minutes and written notification of decisions and recommendations, with the allocated social worker following up to clarify any outstanding issues. Minutes should contain details of who attended, the category under which the child has been registered, the name of the key worker, the unresolved issues of child protection, the interagency work necessary to deal with these, and how the child protection plan is related to the identified needs and risks.

The child

The conference will be convened because of a child needing help and protection and therefore it is essential to remain focused on the needs and, if appropriate, wishes of the child. At the outset of the investigation into an incident or allegation the social worker should be taking account of the ascertainable views of the child. This view should then form a central part of the initial assessment and the report to conference.

On occasion there will be sufficient concerns for a prebirth initial conference to be convened. Such a conference should have the same status and be conducted in exactly the same way as any initial conference, and the child's name may go on the CPR. In the case of an unborn or very young child the mother's needs will sometimes take over and become the centre of attention. On another occasion a particular practitioner may have issues directly or indirectly related to the case in question and the conference may become hijacked. Such circumstances are rare, but the practitioner entering the conference arena for the first time needs to keep them in mind and remain focused on the child even if others around them are not.

If the child is of an appropriate age and development where he or she can and wants to attend the conference then the child should be encouraged to do so. However, if the abuser is also to attend then great care needs to be taken that the abuse does not continue during the conference. This can take many forms, from an abusive parent using direct verbal and physical threats, to more subtle emotional abuse. In our view it should be the parent/abuser who should be refused access to the conference or removed, with the child being given support to stay. The fact that the child is the centre of the process should be clearly demonstrated to everyone. There is also a danger that the conference itself may become abusive if practitioners are indiscriminate with what they say and the chairperson does not manage the meeting with a focus on the needs of the child.

The parents and family

Although the family members are not required to attend the conference by law, it is important they are invited unless there are clear and stated reasons why all or individual family members should be excluded. Parental understanding of concerns, expectations and recommendations arising from the conference can have positive results. Secrecy is where problems can begin and fester, while openness can facilitate a healthy, positive environment in which to work. Parents have a natural right and responsibility to be heard and to hear what is being said about them and their children. There is often concern amongst practitioners that involving parents openly in the process will create conflict. However, not only can parents provide accurate factual information, they will often know the reality of a situation better than anyone even if they do not have insight into its cause or effect. They are uniquely placed to assist the conference. It has already been mentioned in previous chapters that partnership increases parents' confidence in the agencies and the process and it can promote within a parent a greater sense of responsibility towards the child. It may also assist in engaging the family in the detail of the child protection plan, improving relationships between practitioners and families, and increase the chances of successfully protecting the child.

Parents and children should be invited to attend conferences unless the chairperson decides that their exclusion is justified as their attendance would preclude proper consideration of the child's interests. If there is evidence to suggest that the conference may be disrupted because of verbal or physical violence, or because the child will be intimidated, then it is reasonable to exclude the parents. However, the issue should be reassessed at any subsequent conference and the reasons for exclusion should be recorded in the minutes of the meeting.

Locally agreed procedures will outline how child and family attendance at the conference will be managed. Including them in the process reflects the Act's commitment to partnership. It also assists in good practice by requiring practitioners openly to examine envisaged problems with the family. (Local ACPCs should address these issues with practitioners through interagency training and shared policy development.) If parents and children do not attend the conference then the social worker involved must reflect the views of the children and family and these must be recorded in the minutes. However, every effort should be made to get them there and a variety of assistance offered. This can be made available to the family to facilitate their attendance and should not only come from social services but from all the practitioners and agencies involved, and could include the following:

- leaflets, or booklets in a variety of languages and formats explaining the process and purpose of the conference
- financial and practical assistance for family members wishing to attend a conference, such as convenient scheduling, an accessible venue, transport, and childminding or crèche facilities
- giving parents and children the right to bring a 'friend' to support them. It is becoming common practice for parents to bring solicitors. Solicitors have no status at a conference beyond being there to 'support' the parents and are certainly not allowed to attend the conference in order to question anyone there.

Process of the conference and registration

As explained above there are two types of conference, the initial and the review conference. The process for both is similar and the following typical agenda (as recommended in *The Challenge of Partnership in Child Protection: Practice Guide*, DoH 1995) can be used as a model for either:

- introduction of those present
- identification of key people who are absent
- the purposes and objectives of the conference
- the rules of the conference, for example confidentiality, equal opportunities
- verification of details about the family
- presentation of the details surrounding the alleged incident or cause for concern
- presentation of the initial assessment
- the family's perspective on the incident or cause for concern (the child's perspective and the adult's perspective should be given separately)
- presentation of views of family members (including the feelings and wishes of the child) who are not present
- discussion of nature and level of risk to the child
- discussion about the value of registration and its impact on the protection of the child
- decision about registration
- appointment of key worker if registration is agreed
- recommendations to each agency about future action within the child protection system (an outline child protection plan) or through the provision of other services
- date of next review.

For a child to be registered, or remain on the register, the conference must decide that the child is, or is likely to be, at risk of significant harm under one or more of the four categories described in Chapter 5: neglect, physical injury, sexual abuse or emotional abuse. The decision to register should be a result of the information set before the conference and the discussions that follow. It must be based on the needs of the child and be made in the best interests of the child. The actual process by which a conference reaches a decision may be different depending on local procedures. In some places there is a vote, in some a consensus is reached and in others a decision is arrived at through the directions of the chairperson.

Reports

Decisions at the conference must follow from consideration of all the available information that will be contained chiefly in the report prepared by the investigating social worker, but also in written and verbal reports from those other practitioners involved with the family. The social worker's report will include an interagency chronology of recent events, immediate causes for concern, detailed information about the child and if possible the views of the child, a family history including previous contact with relevant agencies, and an appraisal of the family's ability to protect the child and their will-ingness to cooperate with practitioners.

Many areas now have a standard pro forma that gives the investi-gating social worker a guide to layout and topics to be covered in the report, but this can change from area to area or office to office. The most important thing is that the report is child focused and contains the essentials that will allow the conference to make an objective assessment. Whatever form the introductory report takes it should have been discussed with the family - information shared at the confer-ence should not come as a surprise to them. Indeed it is helpful if there is a place on the report for the child and parents to write their own comments. Above all, the child, if appropriate, and family should be invited and their attendance encouraged and made positive.

Apart from the report of the investigating social workers, reports to conference from those practitioners involved with the child and family should be brief and concentrate on relevant information and reflect the needs of the child. Written reports are useful, and should particularly be submitted if a practitioner cannot attend. However, verbal presentations are equally helpful and practitioners involved with the family should make every effort to attend.

The report prepared by the investigating social worker should explain why the conference has been convened, give specific details as to the referral, and outline what has happened during the course of the investigation. This should include an indication of how the family has reacted to the disclosure and investigation and the level of cooperation received from the family during the investigation.

As background there should be an explanation of the family structure and description of the home circumstances. There should also be information about previous contact between the family and the agencies and if the child has been registered or subject to court proceeding in the past. A chronology is especially useful if there is a complicated or disputed sequence of events.

The views and feelings of the child are most important and these should also be contained in the report if the child is of an age when it can voice them. Otherwise the investigating social worker should comment in relation to the child's development. Finally, the social worker should give an opinion as to the type and levels of risk existing as far as the child is concerned.

Confidentiality

The outcome of a child protection investigation depends on the quality and accuracy of the information that is shared by practitioners. This point was emphasised in Chapter 6, reminding practitioners that successful child protection is based a good teamwork between the agencies and that every contribution is important to the whole. Too many investigations have failed to protect children because practitioners have failed or been reluctant to share information. Both the General Medical Council and the United Kingdom Central Council for Nursing, Midwifery and Health Visiting issue codes of conduct for when and how to share confidential information on children and families. *Working Together* and local procedures also confirm the duty of all practitioners to share information when there is reason to believe a child is being abused or is at risk of significant harm.

Information shared with the investigating social worker or during the conference will remain confidential to those involved. Nevertheless, practitioners may be concerned about sharing information that the family will hear. There may be concerns that this will harm the relationship between the practitioner and family or, in rare cases, the practitioner may be worried that a parent may become vengeful. If there are genuine concerns then the practitioner should discuss these with the investigating social worker and/or chairperson of the conference and, if appropriate, the information may be shared between practitioners without the family's knowledge.

Throughout this book there has been an emphasis on the importance of conducting investigations and conferences in as open a manner as possible, explaining that it will in fact assist in protecting the child, working with the family and producing successful outcomes. The sharing of information at a conference should be on a need-to-know basis and the family also needs to know unless explicit reasons can be found for not telling them.

Deregistration and removal of names

Deregistration should be considered at every review conference. Any of the agencies involved with the child may request that a conference is convened to consider the possibility of deregistration. To justify deregistration members of the conference must be satisfied that the abuse or risk of abuse is no longer exists or is no longer significant. This may be true when work has been undertaken to reduce the presenting risk, when the child or abuser has been removed from the abusive situation, or when circumstances have changed significantly resulting in the risk being reduced. If the conference agrees that the child's name should be removed from the register this must be recorded in the minutes.

A child's name will also be removed if the child moves to another area when liaison will take place with the new area. Under these circumstances a child's name will normally be placed on the register of the new area while a review is convened.

Case study 5b

Directly the information about Sharon, Peter and Andrew was received from the hospital the appropriate manager instructed a social worker to begin the relevant checks with social services records and other agencies to see what information could be gleaned about the family. The manager then contacted the police and it was agreed to hold a strategy meeting at the social services office as soon as possible. The meeting took place between the investigating social worker, the police officer and the manager and it was agreed that Sharon should be visited in hospital.

The investigating social worker and a police officer visited Sharon later that morning in hospital. They explained who they were, why they were there and the concerns that had been expressed. At first Sharon was reluctant to talk to them, minimising the issues and on several occasions asking them to leave. However, through gentle discussion Sharon began to acknowledge her own fears for herself and the children and admitted there had been a number of incidents. In particular she was concerned about Sophie, as the child had both been hit by her stepfather and also witnessed domestic violence.

Sharon gave her permission for Sophie to be jointly interviewed and that afternoon Sharon and the investigating officers collected the child from school. The joint interview took place at the local victim examination suite where Sophie was interviewed by the investigating social worker and police officer in the presence of her mother. Both practitioners had been trained in accordance with the *Memorandum of Good Practice* (Home Office/DoH 1992). The interview was videotaped. Sophie was at first reluctant to talk to the interviewers, holding her mother's hand and staring down at the floor. Slowly she began to relax and told them in her own words about being hit by her stepfather and the things she had seen. The domestic violence had especially frightened her as she had been worried for the safety of her mother. Sharon was returned to the hospital to be near the baby and with her agreement the other children were voluntarily accommodated by social services under Section 22 of the Act.

The investigating police officer visited Peter at his place of work unannounced late that afternoon. To begin with Peter was amiable and welcoming. However, as the interview continued and the officer explained what had happened and that the children had been accommodated and Sharon would be remaining in hospital, Peter's attitude changed. He reminded her who he was, that as an 'important' local politician he knew plenty of people and could have her head on a plate if he wanted. Peter became more hostile, his comments infused with sexual innuendo and threat. Eventually the police officer left and returned to the social services office where a further strategy meeting took place. It was agreed that an initial conference would be convened.

The conference took place at the hospital. Peter and Sharon were there with their solicitor, as were representatives from the children's schools, the education welfare officer, the health visitor, the family GP, hospital staff, the investigating social worker, the police officer, the local authorities legal adviser and a minute taker. The NSPCC and probation service had sent their apologies. An experienced female service manager from social services chaired the conference.

The chairperson invited each person to introduce himself or herself and then explained how the conference would operate. She then asked everyone to take a few moments to read the report prepared by the investigating social worker. Peter interrupted, saying that he had read the report prepared by 'that woman' and it was all 'rubbish'. He added that he intended to make a formal complaint. The chairperson confirmed that he of course had that right, but that the conference was there to consider the issues and to focus on the children and that everyone would be given the opportunity to speak. She then invited the investigating social worker to present her report. The report outlined the circumstances that had led to the convening of the conference, family background, information about each of the children and, where appropriate, her views and the apparent risks.

The conference members decided to record all the children's names on the CPR under the category of emotional abuse. This category was chosen as opposed to physical abuse as the conference members felt that it was the emotional environment of the family which constituted the greatest level of significant harm to the children.

Those practitioners who would be working most closely with the family were identified, as were the roles and responsibilities they held in relation to the child protection plan together with the date of the next conference. The social worker was identified as the person responsible for convening a planning meeting with the key practitioners, Sharon and Peter to decide how best to ensure that the children were protected and that the aims and objectives of the child protection plan were achieved by the date of the review conference.

Commentary

The purpose of the conference is to undertake an interagency assessment of the level of risk facing Sophie, Elizabeth and Andrew, decide if that level of risk is sufficient to constitute significant harm, and if so to record the children's names on the CPR and identify a child protection plan or agree that a planning meeting should take place when the plan would be devised.

Chapter 8
Protecting children in the family

Introduction

Chapter 7 dealt with some of the issues and the role of the conference as the interagency forum that underpins child protection work. Prior to that consideration was given to the notion of significant harm, the establishment of which is the criteria for recording a child's name on the CPR under one or more of the four categories. As was pointed out, the decision as to whether significant harm has or is likely to occur is the only decision required to be made at the conference. On other issues practice may vary, such as whether a key worker is allocated to the child at this stage, or whether a child protection plan is identified detailing how the child is to be protected. As far as the conference is concerned the basic decision of whether or not to register is enough. The discussion now moves on to what comes afterwards.

This chapter focuses on the principle protection of children within the family as their parents are likely to be responsible for the child's abuse. It recognises that in order to protect children, practitioners must work in partnership with the child's parents to promote a safe environment for the child, both physical, and psychological.

> A co-operative working relationship between the helping services and families is essential if the welfare of the child is to be ensured. This co-operative relationship is more likely to be achieved if parents are encouraged to take as large a part as possible from the outset in decisions about the protection of their child and the appropriate services need to ensure that the child remains safe. Similarly children are more likely to place their trust in those who keep them fully informed, find sensitive ways of seeking their views, and pay attention to what they say when making plans for their future. (DoH 1995, p. 68)

It also examines the likely outcomes for the child having been involved in the child protection process. The aim of this chapter is to inform the reader and to dispel some of the myths that may exist around the realistic and achievable results from the child's perspective.

The purpose of the following discussion is to take the reader briefly through the process from the initial conference, the identification of the child protection plan, the application of that plan, the practitioners most likely to be involved and finally concluding with the review conference. There is also a brief mention on how the agencies involved can manage the abuser if they have contact with the child. The chapter is written assuming that the child is being cared for at home and that the parents are considered to be the cause of the significant harm the child has suffered or is likely to suffer. It should be remembered that families are constructed in many ways so the term 'family' should not be thought of as necessarily meaning a heterosexual couple with both parents present.

There will also be discussion on the difficulties of working in partnership with parents whilst remaining child focused, and unpicking the aims and objectives of the child protection plan together with the roles and responsibilities of the practitioners involved.

The chapter is divided into four stages according to the nature of the work being undertaken. This is done in an attempt to show the continuity and interdependence of the child protection process from the initial concern through to the identification of an interagency child protection plan. A process that is aimed at moving from what can be felt by the parents as hostile and punitive in the beginning to engagement and empowerment, and the purpose of which is to facilitate the development of the parents' skills in parenting and protecting their child.

Stage 1

As already stated in previous chapters, the process will often begin with a single practitioner, perhaps in A&E, identifying a concern and passing the information on to social services. What follows may appear to hospital-based practitioners as a 'flurry of activity' leading up to the initial conference followed by a period of apparent inactivity. Indeed it is often a failure on the part of social services to inform the initial referrer of outcomes which can lead to a sense of frustration and annoyance in the practitioner, especially as much may actually be happening.

In many ways it can be argued that the first assessment of risk is undertaken by the practitioner who identifies a concern. This is likely, although by no means certain, to be a period that can seem threatening and intimidating from the parents' point of view. In addition, practitioners can feel as though they are taking on a policing role. Indeed this sense can be increased if social services feel the risk is such that a child needs to be removed into local authority care either on a voluntary basis or through the intervention of the courts. This will only be done if there is an evidential risk to the child and even here it is possible to maintain a working partnership with parents that can overcome their understandable anger and fear.

There has been discussion about the difficulty practitioners may have at this time; balancing the need to work in partnership with parents with maintaining the welfare of the child as the paramount consideration. It can feel difficult and uncomfortable for practitioners to discuss concerns openly with parents, however it is essential that this approach is taken as honesty and clarity now will assist the parents to protect their child in the future. Ambiguity and minimisation in an attempt to spare the parents' distress will not help them to begin the process of addressing concerns arising from the care they provide for their child. Neither will it assist in the relationship that the practitioner must establish in order to help them address these concerns. Practitioners who have shared their concern with the parents and who have explained to them why they are contacting the social services will be in a far better position to speak openly when attending the conference. The reason for reminding ourselves of this is to show that from concern to protection is a process consisting of many interlinking elements with each element aimed at building a protective framework around the child with the parents as the providers of that framework. Therefore at each stage that will follow, this must be kept in mind if practitioners are truly to work in partnership to protect the child at risk. At the same time it has to be acknowledged there are times when practitioners should not tell the parents of the referral if the risk to the child might be increased or the practitioner will be put in danger.

Stage 2

This stage of the assessment process is the Section 47 investigation which was discussed in Chapter 4. As with Stage 1 it can be felt by the parents to be frightening and intimidating, with practitioners again feeling as though they are involved in a policing role rather than one of partnership. It remains critical to the safety of the child that all practitioners cooperate, share information, are open and honest with parents and remain child-centred.

As was seen in Chapter 6, collecting the evidence is the responsibility of all child protection practitioners with the investigating social worker acting as the fulcrum in the process. It is at this stage the assessment will begin to clarify the nature of the concerns and the extent of the risk, if any, to the child. It is essential that that those practitioners involved listen to and work with all members of the immediate family and in doing so encourage individuals to focus on the needs and wishes of the child. Parents fail to parent correctly for many reasons and may be unaware of their own abusive behaviour. The more practitioners generate discussion with parents on how things can be improved the greater the chance of successful rehabilitation. The child may still be on the ward during this process and hospital-based practitioners can be an essential part of developing this positive partnership. Discuss issues with the investigating social worker and be prepared to develop a shared approach towards child and parents.

Stage 3

Stage 3 occurs during the conference itself and in many ways can be thought of as the beginning of the empowerment process of the parents. As was discussed in Chapter 7, this is the forum in which all those involved with the child's welfare will be present in order to make the decision as to whether significant harm has occurred or is likely to occur to that child. If the decision is that significant harm has occurred or is likely to occur then the child's name is recorded on the CPR. In order to reach this decision those involved will be required to discuss their concerns in an open and objective way giving their reasons and possible consequences to the child should the identified risks be allowed to continue.

The parent present during this discussion will, quite possibly for the first time, hear the full extent of the harm their child has suffered or is likely to suffer, together with the possible consequences. They will also see the variety of practitioners involved with their child's welfare and the extent of the interagency nature of child protection. Although it may not seem so at the time, being present during such a discussion can begin the process of empowering the parents by giving them a number of key messages, one of which is the extent to which they can be compelled to work with the agencies and the consequences of non-cooperation. Another key message is that it is they who are responsible for their child's protection and that it is they who will be helped and supported to fulfil those responsibilities. With the emphasis of the discussion on the needs of the child, the parents as responsible for their child and the aim of keeping the child in the home, the scene is set for continuing and building on the empowerment of the parents.

Having said this, the difficulties parents may have in hearing concerns about their parenting skills should not be underestimated, as neither should the difficulties some practitioners may feel at being openly critical. However, if managed well this is a powerful forum in which to achieve the immediate and long-term protection of the child through that child's parents.

Stage 4

Stage 4 begins once the decision has been made to record the child's name on the CPR. This is a complex process of working with the family, continuing the assessment and managing the risk to the child and occupies the period of time from the recording of the child's name to the review conference. *Working Together* provides that the review conference should be held no later than six months after the initial one. However in many local authorities this time frame is shortened to three months. It was said in the introduction that local practice may vary as to whether the child's social worker, known as the key worker, is allocated at the conference as may be the practice of identifying the child protection plan. Whatever the local practice, it is vital that a key worker is identified and that a clear plan of how to protect the child exists, something of which the following reminds us:

> Placing a child's name on the register is not a magic spell which thereafter protects the child from evil. It is a way of alerting professionals to the fact that the child is thought to be at risk. (DoH 1990)

In many ways Stages 1, 2 and 3 can be described as the 'tip of the iceberg' as, having identified that the child is at risk, the question to be answered now is how to reduce or remove that risk. *Working Together* states that all children whose names are placed on the child protection register should have their needs comprehensively assessed. It reminds us that once the child's name is recorded a child protection plan should be identified so that a full understanding of the needs of the child and his family can be established, the purpose of which is to provide a sound basis for future decision making. The forum for identifying this plan is usually a planning meeting held a few days after the initial child protection case conference and attended by the key worker, the health visitor, possibly the school nurse, and other practitioners likely to be closely involved with the family during this assessment period. In some areas of the country this group of people is referred to as the core group, with other practitioners identified as taking on more specific aspects of the plan such as paediatric or psychiatric assessment. Hospital-based practitioners may be involved in this way as part of an assessment or treatment process. Practice may vary as to whether the parents are invited to attend, but in any event they will be informed of the contents of the plan together with their involvement and the expectation of them.

Working Together goes on to describe the following nine key areas of consideration when identifying the child protection plan:

1 Who will undertake the assessment?
2 Where will it be undertaken?
3 What is the timescale?
4 How should it be recorded?
5 How will the family be involved?
6 What is the legal status of the child?
7 How will it fit in with any court action, and have the necessary steps in relation to this been taken?
8 How will it fit in with other action, e.g. by the police, in respect of the offence?
9 What is the social services department's position regarding parental responsibility?

Such an assessment should include contributions from all relevant agencies to cover social, environmental, medical and developmental circumstances. Some of the families will be well known to the child protection agencies and it is essential to draw on this information and utilise records to the full. Guidance on an assessment can be found in *Protecting Children: A Guide for Social Workers Undertaking a Comprehensive Assessment* (DoH 1991b: it is often referred to as the orange book literally because of the colour of the cover).

The comprehensive assessment will inform the child protection plan. It will often be the major tool for work with the child and the family who should be encouraged and enabled to participate in the assessment and planning. In addition to this, *Working Together* goes on to emphasise the need for a written child protection plan identifying the roles and responsibilities of the practitioners involved (taking into account their statutory responsibilities), the part the parents will be expected to play (making clear the expectation of them), and the short-, medium- and long-term goals together with possible consequences of any lack of cooperation. It is the key worker who has responsibility for coordinating this plan, pulling together all contributions into a report for discussion at the review conference.

Having discussed in brief the key elements of the child protection plan of which the comprehensive assessment may be a central component, it would be useful to look at the process of the comprehensive assessment itself in a little more detail. It may be helpful to think of Stages 1, 2 and 3 as mostly concerning the decisions that need to be made in the short term with Stage 4 as the long-term and predictive stage. Stage 4 is about the holistic experience of the child: whether that experience is presenting a risk to their health and wellbeing, if so how it can be changed to reduce or minimise that risk, and what is the likelihood of effecting that change in time for the child's developmental needs. In short, Stage 4 is a diagnostic tool the use of which will identify the appropriate treatment.

Risk assessment and management

When thinking of the assessment and management of risk it is helpful to first establish the ultimate objective. In this context the objective is the removal or minimisation of the level of risk to the child, both immediate and long term. In order to achieve this objective the practitioners will need to develop and work to a plan which aims to change the parenting experience of the child. To do this the practitioners must work with the child's parents, who will be expected to achieve the objective that will allow for the removal of their child's name from the CPR.

It is fair to say that this area of work is highly specialised and should be undertaken by experienced practitioners - often drawn from family centres, or the voluntary or independent sector. The practitioner chosen needs to keep in mind the close and interdependent nature of the relationship between the child and the parents as it is this relationship which provides the primary socialisation for the child and therefore their understanding of themselves and those around them. In addition, the assessment will start from the basic assumption that harm has occurred or is likely to occur to the child and the parents are the cause of that harm. The process itself is child-centred, focusing on the needs of the child and how those needs can best be addressed.

The social services in the form of the key worker carries the statutory responsibility for ensuring that this work is undertaken and that the child is protected. This may mean the use of court orders such an interim care order, an assessment order and, if necessary, an emergency protection order. However, the social services do not carry this responsibility alone. As already mentioned the core group is likely to include the family's health visitor, the school nurse and possibly the midwife, with other practitioners involved as necessary. They will be required to work with the family to facilitate the overall objective.

The assessment undertaken need not necessarily be a full comprehensive assessment as described in the orange book, but it is likely to include an assessment of the child's health and wellbeing, their relationship with their parents and siblings together with their position within the overall dynamics of the family. It will include an assessment of the parents, their own experience of being parented, their relationship with their child(ren) and with each other and their parenting skills. It may also include an assessment of their health and wellbeing and the likelihood of them continuing to abuse their child. This can be especially relevant in cases involving sexual abuse when a family member is suspected of being or is known to be the abuser and the ongoing risk they present to the child. There will also be an assessment of the parents' ability to change/develop their parenting skills within a time frame consistent with the child's developmental needs.

As mentioned earlier, *Working Together* states that a child whose name is recorded on the CPR should have a review of that registration at intervals no longer that six months apart, although in many local authority areas this is undertaken every three months in the form of a review conference. It is at this review that the relevant members of the agencies involved discuss the outcome of the assessment with a view to deciding on the need to maintain the child's name on the CPR. The criteria upon which this will be based are the same as that of the initial conference, i.e. the existence of actual or potential significant harm. However, this decision will in many ways be far more complex process than that of the initial conference. By the time of the review conference a great deal of information will have been obtained as a result of the assessment which will need to be taken into account. Bearing in mind the purpose of the CPR as a means of alerting agencies that a child is at risk, this decision, together with the information which informs that decision, underpins the continued protection of the child. A decision to remove the child's name will remove the means of identifying the child at risk. A decision to continue registration longer than is necessary can undermine the progress made by the parents with a variety of consequences such as a withdrawal of cooperation, a loss of their self-esteem and so on. However, a decision to deregister too early can put the child at risk by virtue of their reduced visibility. Should abuse be subsequently suspected or detected the process will begin again.

Abuser management

Abusers do not go away; they remain in the imagination of the victim and often they continue to be a physical and emotional force not only in the life of the victim and the family but also as far as the practitioners involved are concerned. Their presence may not intrude into the protection plan, if for instance they are given a long custodial sentence, or they may become the major factor if they are a member of the family. A development that has grown from the progress made in interagency child protection has been the growth in interagency offender management in the sharing of information, assessments and treatment projects. This has in part arisen from the acknowledgement that if the objective of all plans is to rehabilitate children back into the family practitioners need at the same time to be addressing the behaviour of the abuser. Most families want to stay together and the majority of parents who abuse will be willing to cooperate by working on their own behaviour.

This may take many forms, from parents receiving assistance with their parenting skills to anger management and sex offender treatment programmes. The progress made by the parents or individual on any of these will be fed into the assessment and influence the plan for keeping the child safe. If an abuser is sent into custody then depending on the length of sentence and prison allocated they may have access to similar programmes, attendance at which may help with early release on licence. The prison will inform the local authority when an inmate is about to be released and strategy meetings or conferences may be organised in response. Abuser management is a growing part of the overall child protection process.

Case study 5c

The planning meeting took place five days after the conference at which Andrew, Sophie and Elizabeth's names had been registered under the category of emotional abuse. Despite threats from Peter to stay away, both Sharon and he attended. Their solicitor did not. Peter had been given an official caution for striking Sophie. The investigating social worker and the health visitor had met with the family between times; both had emphasised the importance of working together to reduce the risk to the children. The investigating social worker had also introduced a colleague for the 'long term' who would be working with the family after the planning meeting. Both Peter and Sharon were pleased that the investigating social worker was being replaced, appearing to see her replacement as a 'softer option'. Peter remained resentful, but appeared to at least recognise the inevitability of the situation when he told the social worker that 'the quicker we get this sorted, the quicker we get rid of you'.

The practitioners immediately involved with the family were invited to the planning meeting, as was a representative from the NSPCC. The atmosphere was relaxed compared with the tensions of the conference. A social services manager chaired the meeting and briefly explained why they were there and the investigating social worker gave a brief update before outlining the areas of concern. The meeting then discussed how these concerns might be met, involving Sharon and Peter as much as possible.

The plan contained the following elements:

- a comprehensive assessment to be prepared by two workers from the NSPCC
- Sharon would attend the mother and baby drop-in group at the family centre every Wednesday and a sessional worker from the family centre would offer to work with Peter on anger management
- the health visitor would continue to visit and make a referral to child and family therapy
- the schools would continue to monitor the progress of the children
- the allocated social worker would visit the family weekly and coordinate the services going into the family from the other agencies.

Three months later the comprehensive assessment prepared by the NSPCC was presented to a further planning meeting. In general the assessment was optimistic, suggesting that the risk of significant harm had greatly reduced and that, as long as the family continued to work with the agencies involved, this would continue to be so. The others involved all reported progress. The family centre sessional worker said that Peter was still prone to angry outbursts, but that they were looking at strategies for Peter to adopt to avoid taking these out on Sharon or the children.

Three months after the initial conference the review conference deregistered the children. Although some concerns still existed about Peter's attitude towards women and his ability to control his temper, it was felt that the risk had been reduced to a point that meant registration was no longer necessary. However, it was recognised that the family still needed to work with the various agencies involved with the family and that if concerns were raised again an initial conference could be convened.

Chapter 9
The court arena

Introduction

Here is a straightforward account of what the doctor or nurse can expect once involved in the court arena. This will be a rare event, often only involving 'expert' medical practitioners, but it is useful for all practitioners involved in child protection to have some knowledge of each stage of the process. A distinction is drawn between family and criminal proceedings, explaining the purpose and difference between the two together with the likely experience of appearing as an expert witness. The chapter does not attempt to go into any great detail about either the civil or criminal court, but instead gives an impression of how they operate, the powers they have and, in the case of the criminal court, possible outcomes and how these may affect the child protection process.

In any court case involving a child, be it in the civil or criminal court, there are two clocks ticking; first the adult or court clock that reflects standard time, and second the child's clock which will often be running in accordance with the particular child's development. The younger the child the quicker this developmental clock will run, demanding that the court reach as swift a decision as it is able. In civil proceedings the Act has gone some way to ensure that the family court recognises the developmental needs of the child, and that delay for even a few weeks can result in significant harm or impairment. As shall be seen, the directions hearing is used to enable speedy proceedings and make certain that progress is being made in the interests of the child. The adult criminal court, however, remains a far more ponderous animal where the needs and feelings of child victims, often to be called as witnesses, are not the priority.

The courts and court practitioner

In civil proceedings the Act created a unified structure with three levels for cases involving children and families as follows:

* family proceedings court.
* county court
* family division of the High court.

Childcare cases are initiated in the family proceedings court presided over by magistrates who should be experienced in dealing with cases involving children and families. If the case is deemed to be too complicated or contentious then it will be transferred to the county court where it will be heard by a single judge. An application to transfer can be made by any of the parties. This may happen, for instance, when there is a complex medical diagnosis involved in the case and both sides may be calling 'expert' witnesses with conflicting views. Moving cases between courts can increase the length of time spent in proceedings, something the Act has sought to reduce.

In criminal proceedings all adults charged with a criminal offence will be first dealt with in the magistrates' court in front of two or three lay magistrates, or a single legally qualified stipendiary magistrate. The majority of adult criminal cases are dealt with at this level, but serious crimes, for which the magistrates do not have the required breadth of sentencing powers, will be sent to the Crown Court. Criminal cases involving young people under the age of 18 will begin in the youth court, but may be transferred to the Crown Court depending on their seriousness. The Crown Court is presided over by a judge with a jury if there is a not guilty plea to be heard. Appeals are heard in the Crown Court from the magistrates and in the High Court from the Crown Court. Adults charged with offences against children may be heard in either depending upon the seriousness of the charge.

The Act recognises the need to avoid delay in order that the child's welfare should not suffer and has introduced directions appointments to assist in ensuring that the case is heard as quickly as possible. This allows the parties and the court to timetable the proceedings, to make certain that statements and plans are ready, witnesses available and that all those involved are remaining focused on the child. There can be more that one directions appointment. The *guardian ad litem* (GAL) will be central to these proceedings representing the needs and wishes of the child.

The GAL is an independent social worker appointed by the court to represent the child during court proceedings. Since 1984 the courts have been required to appoint GALs from panels established by local authorities in accordance with regulations made under the Children Act 1975. The Act further enhanced the role of the GAL. The GAL has access to the individuals and documents involved in the case. The GAL may call for their own independent reports or 'expert' witnesses and will be represented by their own solicitor, who will also act for the child unless the child disagrees with the GAL, in which case the GAL will find another solicitor.

In civil proceedings the social services department will be advised, supported and represented in civil proceedings by the local authority's legal advisers. Arrangements for these legal services will differ between authorities, with some retaining an in-house legal team while others place most or all legal work out to competitive tender. If the service is in-house then the department will be staffed by solicitors and possibly barristers with childcare expertise and will be able to employ other legal representatives on a case-by-case basis as consultants or to represent the authority in court. Otherwise cases will be allocated to solicitors in private practice on a case-by-case basis. In criminal cases the Crown Prosecution Service (CPS) will conduct the prosecution, again either using in-house solicitors or assigning casework to local solicitors at a magistrates' court and hiring barristers for the Crown Court. The parents of a child or the defendant in a criminal case will have to find their own legal representative. In most areas there will be a list of specialist childcare solicitors available. Qualification for legal aid is dependent on the circumstances of the individual, but parents would normally expect to get assistance if their means were not adequate to cover the costs of court action.

Medical evidence

This chapter does not concern itself in detail with the use, presentation and significance of medical evidence in court, but it is appropriate to mention briefly when and how it might be used and to remind readers that clinicians can carry significant authority within the court setting. Medical evidence may be used in magistrates', Crown and civil courts and will usually fall into one of the following categories: as a police statement, for inclusion in the statement of a social worker, as 'expert' testimony, or another party to the proceedings.

In a criminal investigation into a case of child abuse, the police may wish to take a statement from any practitioner involved in the case, such as a triage nurse in A&E who first treated the child. This will be in the form of a witness statement. As highlighted in the chapter on collecting the evidence it is vitally important for practitioners to base what they say on what they know to have happened and to be objective. It does not follow that having given a statement that the case will go to prosecution or that they will be asked to attend court. It is important that if they have any concerns, or doubts about this process that they consult their relevant line manager.

Later in this chapter the role of the social services during care proceedings is discussed and mention is made of the statements and reports that may be prepared in support of a particular application. One of the most important will be the initial statement of evidence that the social worker making the application to court has to submit. In this report the social worker will outline the concerns and reasons for making the application and may mention information gleaned from a number of sources to support the case. This may include information gathered from nursing or medical practitioners either directly by the social worker or taken from social services files. The social worker must be circumspect in using this information, using it to support the main thrust of the argument rather than presenting it as evidence-in-chief. Medical practitioners should be aware that information shared with social services might be later used in this way. This should not make them wary or hesitant, but encourage them to make certain information is correct.

While most nursing and medical practitioners will not have actually to appear in court, doctors are instructed to prepare court reports and appear as witnesses for magistrates', Crown and civil courts. In these cases the practitioner would normally be regarded as an 'expert' witness. Under the Rules of Evidence a lay witness may only comment on fact as they know it, but an 'expert' may also give opinion. The 'expert' will often be required to give a view on issues beyond the specific individual or incident involved; for instance in child protection proceeding the 'expert' may be asked to give an explanation on child development, behaviour and such like in order for the court to place a particular child or event in context.

In a criminal case the defence, prosecution or the court itself may instruct an 'expert'. Medical evidence will usually be requested concerning the offender after conviction, although it may be called upon pre-sentence to address legal matters such as diminished responsibility and recommendations under the Criminal Procedure (Insanity and Unfitness to Plead) Act 1991. A medical report from a psychologist or psychiatrist may also be requested to support a recommendation for a convicted abuser to attend a community-based sex offender treatment programme.

In the family court arena any of the parties, individually or jointly, or the court may request an 'expert' or independent report. Indeed, in childcare cases it is common for the local authority, the GAL and the parents' representative to agree upon a single instruction for an independent report. Equally parties may call their own 'expert', although the court will hope to avoid family court action becoming extended or adversarial and to avoid a plethora of 'experts' becoming involved. Medical evidence may be called upon by the local authority in support of an application for an interim or full care order either because a medical referral has initiated an investigation or assessment, or because the local authority require medical evidence to support their own view.

- In the first instance a paediatrician might refer a child to social services with suspected psychosocial dwarfism after all other medical diagnoses have been ruled out. The social services will then investigate and may discover levels of neglect that support the paediatrician's view that will lead to court action in which the medical view will be pivotal. Likewise, if an A&E unit have reported a non-accidental fracture or other injury then the medical evidence will be essential to any local authority application to court.
- In a second example the social services department may be concerned about parental ability to cope and care correctly for a child and a medical opinion may be sought in order to enhance the social worker's assessment. Equally a child may be referred to local psychiatric services with behavioural, social or emotional difficulties or a delay in development and a report may then be required for court.

By whichever means and to whichever court practitioners give evidence it is important to do so and to retain a clear objectivity in the information given. Decisions of the court will only be as good as the evidence placed before them. If practitioners have any doubts about procedures, the contents of reports or their role in court they should consult with appropriate colleagues. If nervous about going to court, take the opportunity to arrange to visit the court before the hearing and discuss with the other practitioners involved what is likely to happen.

Family proceedings

In Chapter 2, on the legal framework, an outline of the legislation that impinges on childcare was given and in particular the Act was examined as well as the very significant changes it has brought to family court proceedings. It has been explained that the Act encourages negotiation and cooperation between parents, children and practitioners, which it is hoped will enable children to remain within their own families with appropriate intervention and support. The 'no order principle' places the emphasis on the need to work without the use of court orders. However, there are situations when it is necessary to take action through the court in order to protect a child from harm. The Act has given us a range of graduated options.

The Act designates relevant applications as 'family proceedings'. Not all of these are actually written into the Act itself. Some arise from earlier legislation such as the Adoption Act and Domestic Violence and Matrimonial Proceedings Act, both 1976, or since, such as the Human Fertilisation and Embryology Act 1990 and the Family Homes and Domestic Violence Act 1995. It is felt that together they form a raft of legislation that may affect children and therefore come under the umbrella of the term 'family proceedings'. Applications in family proceedings divide into two types: public law applications and private law applications. The first includes emergency protection orders (EPOs) and care orders and the second residence orders and contact orders. At the end of this section brief details are given of each, but here emphasis will be placed on the application for a care order which, along with an EPO, is the one a hospital-based practitioner is most likely to be involved with.

Court action will always be a possible outcome to any child protection investigation or assessment, but it is not always possible to plan ahead, or foresee a change in circumstances. A new referral can warrant immediate action if it is felt a child is at risk and an EPO can be applied for, or a child can be placed under police protection. Both of these actions will keep the child safe and allow the social services department time to undertake an assessment of the situation before taking further court action in the form of an application for an interim or full care order. Staff in A&E and on the ward may have to involve the police in keeping or protecting a child, or preventing a parent from removing a child while he is receiving treatment, and

police protection or an EPO may be used to do this. In Chapter 3
the role of the police and their powers in child protection were examined and here consideration is given to the EPO.

Anyone may apply for an EPO, including, therefore, a medical
practitioner, but usually it will be the local authority or the police,
although the police will usually rely on their Section 46 powers and
the local authority will deal with an EPO application to carry the
matter forward. Before granting an EPO the court have to be satisfied that there is reasonable cause to believe that a child is suffering
or likely to suffer significant harm unless removed from the current
accommodation or if not kept where he or she is, such as in a neona-
tal ward after a premature birth. Social services can also apply for an
EPO if during a Section 47 child protection investigation they
cannot gain access to a child who might be suffering significant
harm. The order initially lasts a maximum of eight days, with the
possibility of a further extension of up to seven days. Because of its
nature it may be granted without notice and by a single justice and
there is no appeal. On application for an emergency protection
order the court appoints a GAL for the child. The order is very
much a temporary or transitional measure and the applicant gains
limited parental responsibility for the child, who may be looked after
in local authority accommodation, hospital or appropriate facility.

The social services will apply for a care order if it believes the
child concerned is suffering from or likely to suffer from significant
harm because the child's parents are unable to care for him or her in
a reasonable way. It is usual for social services to first apply for an
interim care order that may last for an initial eight week period, with
one or more four week extensions available on application. Eight
and four weeks are maximum periods. An interim order allows social
services to further assess the situation while keeping the child safe. A
decision can then be made as to the need to apply for a full care
order. The making of a care order is the only way in which a child
can be taken into the statutory care of a local authority on a long-
term basis. The care order may last until a child reaches 18 or be
discharged earlier on application to the court. A child taken into the
care of the local authority may be later placed for adoption. If this is
the intention of social services then it must be contained in the care
plan presented to the court prior to the hearing.

The care plan is of vital importance because it sets out for the
court and the parties involved how the child is to be cared for, what
contact is planned between the child and the family, how the child is
to be educated and so forth. It will also, as stated above, set out the

final intention of social services as far as long-term care of the child is concerned. This care plan is prepared by the social worker involved. The social worker will also have submitted a chronology, his or her own statement(s) of evidence in support of the application and organised the statements of others such as a health practitioner with particular knowledge of the child or family.

Under the Act there are a range of options open to social services and the family if court action is deemed to be the chosen way forward. Below is a brief explanation of the orders that are available. First, the public law orders:

- *Emergency protection order*: see above.
- *Interim care order* and *care order*: see above.
- *Interim supervision order* and *supervision order*: under Section 31 of the Act the local authority can apply for a supervision order. This acknowledges that the child is at risk of significant harm as with a care order, but the local authority does not seek parental responsibility which remains with the parents.
- *Child assessment order*: this order will be applied for under Section 43 of the Act when social services are frustrated in their attempts to have an assessment undertaken because of a lack of cooperation or resistance from the parents. If the child is thought to be at risk of significant harm but in no immediate danger, then this order may be appropriate. The local authority may apply for this order and all parties will attend court before it is granted. The court will be informed of previous failed attempts to undertake the assessment and be satisfied the order is necessary for the child's welfare. The order may last for up to seven days, during which the child can be removed from home, but it is normally expected that the making of the order will encourage the parents to cooperate and allow the assessment to take place.

The Act also introduced four new orders (collectively known as Section 8 orders) which provide the means for parents and others to resolve disputes about a child's care. Provided the court believes that judicial interference is warranted then all courts in private or public proceedings are able to make one or more of the following orders. Such orders are often made without the local authority becoming involved.

- *Residence order*: this order applies to the person with whom a child will reside and will also cancel any existing care order. It is usually granted to an immediate family member, a parent or grandparent, and can be shared. Parental responsibility may be given with the order to those who do not otherwise have it. For example a grandparent may apply for a residence order if they feel the new partner of their daughter is unsuitable and may place the child at risk of significant harm.

- *Contact order*: this stipulates what contact and access may take place between an adult and child. Contact includes telephone calls, e-mail, Internet communication, tape and video recordings, letters, parcels and any other form of communication that might take place between the child and the adult concerned. Denying contact can be achieved by a prohibited steps order, or an order for no contact in a contact order.
- *Specific issue order*: as the name implies this order is designed to resolve disputes between those with decision-making power in a child's life. For example a local authority, or anyone with leave from the court, may use this provision to seek a ruling from the court on allowing a child medical treatment. Application for a specific issue order to the High Court will be used when a parent refuses to allow medical treatment which medical experts consider necessary in the interests of the child.
- *Prohibited steps order*: like an injunction this order is used to prevent a parent, or someone with parental responsibility, from taking action that is deemed harmful to the child's welfare. It may be obtained in emergencies without notice.

Criminal proceedings

In simple terms the police and CPS want to convict an offender and the social services want to prevent further harm coming to the child. In criminal proceedings the aim is to prove someone guilty of a particular act, such as a sexual assault, while in civil proceedings there is essentially the need only to show that a child is at risk of significant harm and that the parent is unable to protect that child. It is not necessary to identify an individual or prove someone directly responsible for the abuse. For instance, a child may have suffered a non-accidental injury such as a spiral fracture of the arm, responsibility for which it is unclear. No one is taking responsibility and a number of 'suspects' may exist, but the child has to be protected. Social services may therefore proceed to court on the grounds that because the event evidently happened and there is no clear perpetrator, legal action is necessary to protect the child from further harm. It is enough therefore to have evidence to show that harm has taken place.

Criminal and civil cases may be run in tandem with the offender appearing in the criminal court while the child may be subject to proceedings in the civil court. The Act has done much to improve the civil court process in respect of children, moving us towards a system in which the needs of the child are seen to be paramount, yet because of its different nature the criminal system remains far from child friendly.

If child protection is about anything it is about placing the child above and beyond other considerations, of making certain the child is safe, well cared for and, if possible, ultimately happy. Directly one enters the criminal justice system these essential aims may become distorted and there is an ever-present danger that the system may further abuse the child. The British criminal justice system is adversarial and does not fit easily with the needs of the child; indeed the court is there as much to protect the alleged offender as to defend the victim. During the course of such a process the child is therefore vulnerable.

However, if practitioners are to prevent abuse, and child protection has to be about prevention if it has reason beyond being a purely reactive mechanism, then society has also to catch and punish the perpetrator. In doing so the authorities not only impede his or her abusive progress and send a warning to others, but perhaps most importantly it is a clear statement of intent to the victim. It is important for many victims to see their abuser brought to justice. This may not mean sending someone to prison, but punishment acknowledges what has been done, shows it to be true and hopefully begins a journey of regeneration for both victim and offender. If the offence has taken place within the family then this process has added significance.

Successfully punishing the offender is easier said than done and it is a matter of experience that only a small percentage of those who abuse children actually get to court let alone are convicted. As with any criminal case, unless you have an unquestionable confession, gaining a conviction rests with the quality of the evidence. In Chapter 6 it was demonstrated that in a case involving a child victim the body of evidence may be based on nothing greater than what the child has said. In some cases there may be forensic evidence to support this, or the corroborative evidence of a witness, although such information will tend to be regarded as secondary to the evidence given by the child. Whatever the evidential combination it is the mind and body of the child that will hold the key to a successful conviction.

It is vital to remember that the criminal justice system has a primary duty to safeguard the rights of the defendant and as such is not there to protect children. Criminal proceedings will often appear to be at odds with the best interests of a child. There appears to be a stark contrast between the careful sensitivity shown by police and social services staff when conducting a joint interview to obtain video evidence and the often aggressive questioning the same child may experience in court. Likewise the Act has placed an emphasis on abolishing delay, and yet the criminal justice system can be ponderous.

Child witnesses

During recent years there have been changes within the criminal system based on the gradual acceptance that children have an equal right to be heard within the court arena. In 1988 the Criminal Justice Act took a significant step in justice for children by abolishing the assumption that a child was an 'incompetent' witness and making it possible for children to give evidence through the use of television links. The 1991 Criminal Justice Act put an end to the right of the accused to cross-examine the child and allow a video-recorded interview to stand as evidence in chief. In Chapter 6 it was discussed that The Home Office and Department of Health jointly published the *Memorandum of Good Practice* in 1992 which gives professional guidance to those interviewing children to obtain evidence for court.

At the present time there is no national standard to which courts have to adhere, which means that children are treated differently depending on the court in which they are appearing as a witness. Not all courtrooms have video links, some invariably allow the use of video evidence, others expect older children to appear in the witness box where there might or might not be a screen to shield them. Government has been slow to respond to the needs of children appearing as witnesses despite the fact that the difficulties children experience have been well recorded for many years. In 1995 the NSPCC, as part of their continuing Justice for Children campaign, highlighted the trauma children experience through attending court, which some observers have suggested is worse than the original abuse. This view may not only lead children and parents to refuse to be part of court action, but may discourage practitioners from reporting disclosure or actively pursuing cases. An experienced abuser may use the threat of a long drawn-out court case to dissuade his victim, or victim's family, from action.

In June 1998 the Home Office published *Speaking Up for Justice*, a report containing 70 recommendations to improve the treatment not only of child witnesses, but all vulnerable witnesses. However, as with changes in the way adult rape victims can be treated in court, it is unlikely that these recommendations will quickly come into standard practice or that all the suggestions will be taken up. The 1989 Piggot Report (Home Office 1989) made similar recommendations and yet a significant number of these have not been implemented. The crux of the problem appears to be the need to balance the needs of the child victim against the fundamental right of the accused to a fair trial in which he is assumed innocent until found guilty beyond reasonable doubt. While society persists with the current adversarial system this dilemma will remain and a delicate balancing act will be required and justice will have to rely on best practice and a steadily growing awareness amongst court practitioners.

It is hard enough for adults to enter a criminal court as a witness, for a child one can only imagine the anxiety and fear before and during the experience. There is no ideal situation, but best practice would suggest that the child should remain in a separate room from the main court with a 'supporter' with whom the child feels at ease. The room is then linked to the courtroom by way of a video system allowing the jury to watch the child's evidence and the defence to undertake cross-examination. The Judge, prosecution and defence barristers should be child focused in their questioning, although this is not always the case. One can understand the defence cross-examination being robust, but judges sometimes appear unable or unwilling to protect the child when cross-examination becomes too aggressive.

In some courts there are witness-support schemes which provide services to children. The child may be invited to visit the court before the case, be given books, encouraged to play board games depicting court procedures, to dress up like a judge and so forth in an effort to reduce the uncertainty that is related to a court appearance. The child must not be coached or assisted in any way as to how he might give evidence or what he might say.

As a practitioner the essential thing is to support the child, recognising his needs and wishes, but at the same time being aware of the need to protect him and others from future abuse. To do this society must prosecute and convict offenders not so much to punish them, although this is important as far as the Rule of Law and deterrents are concerned, but most importantly to break the cycle of abuse. It is important to recognise the potential difficulties that can exist for practitioners, but also to stress that the level of damage to the child can grow significantly greater if the disclosure or injury is not investigated fully.

The offender

While it is not within the specific remit of this book to examine sentencing and what may happen to individuals found guilty of offences against children it is important to touch upon the subject in order to remind ourselves that offenders do get released or not sent to prison in the first place, often returning into their own communities perhaps to live with or near the original victim. They also continue to present a risk. In the introduction we referred to recent media and public reaction to the dangers, real and imagined, that offenders against children may present and it is vital to bring an objective appraisal to this debate. It is also important to remember that not all offenders against children are sex offenders, that to abandon, neglect or injure a child is also a serious offence and will probably attract the label of Schedule 1. This is applied to anyone committing a specific offence against a child.

The Sex Offender Act 1997 established the sex offender register and guidance has been issued to the police on how the information contained on the register should be handled. Many ACPCs have already established means of exchanging information about sex offenders who pose a risk to children. Prisons are already obliged to inform social services of the imminent release of Schedule 1 offenders into the local community. Sex offender awareness and the political need to respond to public and media pressure has resulted in a demand for in particular social services, the police and probation to increase the amount of resources being spent on tracking, discussing, working with and monitoring sex offenders.

Not all offenders are sent to prison - many will receive sentences that may to the public appear 'light' such as a fine or conditional discharge, while some may be placed on probation. As has already been mentioned the probation service, in partnership with other agencies, runs specific projects for working with dangerous offenders in the community in an attempt to manage the offenders better and reduce the risk to children by influencing the offenders' behaviour.

Information about sentencing is shared between the agencies and strategy discussions will be held if an offender again presents a risk to his original victim or to other children. For instance, a case conference may be called when an offender is about to be released from prison to live with a partner he has met during his sentence and where there are children in the household. A child or children may be placed on the CPR if it is felt this individual will present a risk.

The most important duty for the police is protecting the public, yet the police involvement with violent and dangerous offenders has tended to cease at the point of arrest. Arrest and conviction are only the opening steps in trying to manage an offender's behaviour and protecting children. It is vital that the interagency network continues to exchange information.

Below are listed the most significant offences against a child for which an adult can be charged.

- *Abduction.* The Child Abduction Act 1984, as amended under the Children Act 1989, creates two separate offences against children under the age of 16 years. The first offence (Section 1) may be committed only by a person 'connected with' the child who takes or sends the child out of the UK 'without the appropriate consent', e.g. of the child's parent(s). In the case of a child whose parents were not married at the time a man in respect of whom there are reasonable grounds to believe him to be the father, a guardian, a person in whose favour a residence order is in force with respect to the child or a person having custody. The 'appropriate consent' refers to that of the child's mother, child's father if he has parental responsibility, anyone who has a residence order, any person having custody or the leave of the court under the Act, or in the case of any person having custody, the leave of the court which awarded custody. The second offence (S.2) is committed where a person who is not the child's mother, or where the parents were married at the time of the birth the child's father, or guardian, custodian or a person in whose favour a residence order is in force, without lawful authority or reasonable excuse, takes or detains the child: 1) so as to remove him from the lawful control of any person having lawful control of him; or 2) so as to keep him out of the lawful control of any person entitled to lawful control of him. The maximum sentence on summary conviction (i.e. by magistrates' court) is six months imprisonment and/or a fine, and on indictment (i.e. in a Crown Court) by imprisonment for seven years.
- *Assault occasioning actual bodily harm.* This comes under the Offences Against the Persons Act 1861 as amended (various Acts). Bodily harm needs no explanation according to the House of Lords (Director of Public Prosecutions v Smith 1961).

- *Wounding and grievous bodily harm.* This also comes under the Offences Against the Persons Act 1861 as amended (various Acts): 'Who so ever shall unlawfully and maliciously by any means what so ever wound or cause any grievous bodily harm to any person with intent to resist to or prevent the lawful apprehension of any person shall be guilty of (an offence triable on indictment) and being convicted thereof shall be liable to imprisonment for life' (S.20); 'Who so ever shall unlawfully and maliciously wound or inflict any grievous bodily harm upon any person either with or without any weapon or instrument shall be guilty (of an offence triable either way) and being convicted thereof shall be liable to imprisonment for five years' (S.20). Grievous means 'no more and no less than really serious'.
- *Common assault.* Under the Criminal Justice Act 1988, common assault and battery is a summary offence with a maximum sentence of six months' imprisonment and/or a fine.
- *Concealment of birth.* The Offences Against the Persons Act 1861, as amended, applies to any child alive or dead whose body is disposed of to conceal his birth. It is triable either way (i.e. in a magistrates' or Crown Court) and carries a maximum sentence of two years' imprisonment.
- *Infanticide.* The Infanticide Act 1938 applies to a woman who causes the death of her child in the first twelve months of his life. She can be charged with infanticide rather than murder or manslaughter if found to be suffering from mental illness associated with childbirth. It is triable on indictment and carries a maximum sentence of five years imprisonment.
- *Murder.* Murder is an offence at common law. Is triable on indictment and carries a mandatory life sentence. Under the Criminal Justice Act 1995 it is again triable on indictment - a judge imposing a discretionary life sentence may, as part of the sentence, specify the tariff period. When that period has been served it will be the duty of the Home Secretary to release the prisoner on licence if the parole board agrees.
- *Neglect.* It is offence to assault, ill treat, neglect or abandon a child (under 16) in a manner likely to cause unnecessary suffering or injury to health. The maximum sentence for this offence is 10 years' imprisonment (Children and Young Persons Act 1933 as amended).

Sex offences

- *Rape.* Rape is non-consenting sexual intercourse and it is not necessary for intercourse to be completed; penetration to any degree is sufficient to bring a charge of rape (S.1(1) Sexual Offences Act 1956 as amended by Sexual Offences (Amendment) Act 1976).
- *Incest.* Until the turn of the century this was an ecclesiastical offence, tried by a church court. It is sexual intercourse between certain related persons. Consent is immaterial whatever the age of the victim. It is committed by a man who has intercourse with a woman he knows to be his daughter, granddaughter, mother or sister (including half-sister), and by a woman over 16 who has intercourse with a man she knows to be her father, grandfather, son, brother (or half-brother) (S.10 and S.11, Sexual Offences Act 1956). It is also an offence for a man to incite a girl under 16 to have incestuous sexual intercourse with him (S.54, Criminal Law Act 1977).
- *Buggery.* Like rape, full penetration is not necessary for the offence to be buggery (S.12, Sexual Offences Act 1956 as amended by Sexual Offences Act 1967). Assault with intent to commit buggery is an alternative offence under S.16 of the Act, where an attempt to commit buggery can be proven.
- *Unlawful sexual intercourse (USI).* It is an offence for a man to have intercourse with a girl under 16 to whom he is not married. There is a defence if the victim is aged between 14 and 16, where there is a marriage invalid under English Law, the man is under 24, has not previously been charged with a similar offence and reasonably believes the girl to be over 16 (S.5 and S.6, Sexual Offences Act 1956).
- *Gross indecency.* This offence refers to acts of indecency between males only. Physical contact is not always necessary, for instance to masturbate in public would be an act of gross indecency as would mutual masturbation. Offences include committing an act of gross indecency, being party to the commission, or procuring the commission of the act (S.13, Sexual Offences Act 1956 as amended by Sexual Offences Act 1967).
- *Indecent assault.* There is no clear definition of this offence in law, but there has to be force, or a hostile act accompanied by indecency, for instance an adult might touch a child while suggesting an indecent act (S.14 and S.15, Sexual Offences Act 1956).

- *Indecent conduct with or towards a child.* This can be committed by any person who commits an act of indecency with or towards a child under 14 or who incites a child under 14 to commit such an act. For instance, an adult could be charged with this if he asks a child to perform an indecent act on him, or encourages two children to perform indecent acts on each other providing one child is under 14 (S.1, Indecency with Children Act 1960)
- *Causing or encouraging prostitution or intercourse with or indecent assault on a girl under 16.* The person committing the offence will have responsibility for the girl. It is sufficient for the responsible person to allow the girl to consort with or enter into or continue in the employment of a prostitute or person of known immoral character. The implication is that the person must have knowledge of or allow the action to continue (S. 28, Sexual Offences Act 1956).
- *Indecent photographs of children.* It is an offence for a person to take or allow to be taken or to have in their possession indecent photographs or films of children or to distribute or show them. This may also be applied to activities on the Internet (S.1, Protection of Children Act 1978).

Conclusion

In the introduction, it was stated that the concluding part of this book would be used to debate with the reader some of the more salient issues in relation to the complexities of interagency working for the protection of vulnerable children. By its nature this will be a mechanism of sharing thoughts that have developed as a result of observing the child protection process from a number of different perspectives. Some of what has been seen has been good, some not so good and at times quite frankly some has been poor when seen from the point of view of and consequences to the child concerned. This section is also used as an opportunity to debate with the reader some of the more topical issues around at the time of writing.

The discussion is divided into a number of separate topics concluding with some more general comments in relation to the current political and economic climate in which practitioners work. There is no intent to impart individual political preferences, but simply to translate the possible effects of various messages into the more realistic setting of everyday practice.

Child protection and children in need - the refocusing debate

Paul Boateng has already made his intention and that of the government clear; that society needs to look again at the way it employs social services. The word 'holistic' has appeared in relation to the government's belief that the most vulnerable children and families in our community need help before the dynamics within the family reach a point where a child is abused and a child protection investigation is necessary. There is no doubt that all practitioners would welcome the opportunity to be able to offer preventative work and by this means reduce the amount of child protection currently undertaken. It may be argued that there has been a return to the immediate postwar era, if not before, when agencies treated the symptoms and not the need. Yet to achieve a change, to move in a new direction would require a major change of emphasis in the current delivery of services.

The recent local government reorganisation has created many problems within local authorities, in many parts of the country the county structure for the ACPC has been subdivided into two, three or even more areas with the inevitably negative effect on service provision.

Social services childcare departments currently spend a considerable portion of their budgets on post-abuse child protection activity. One only has to spend a few hours with a children and families duty (reception and assessment) team to see how resources have to be channelled into child protection, leaving little spare for preventative work. Many referrals to the duty teams will be dealt with there or refused a service which means that long-term teams are picking up cases that will inevitably contain a disproportionate number of children already on the CPR or close to being placed there. This also creates the situation in which a comparatively small number of cases are actually being worked, that less demanding cases receive little or no input, that preventative work attracts little attention and that the level of stress and risk under which the staff are working is constantly high.

The scenario described above relates to social services but, with the change of a few words, could easily be relevant to the majority of services called upon to work with children and families. The NHS in its fiftieth year is an example that practitioners can all take considerable pride in the fact, as in all public services, that success has been dependent on many things, such as policy making, funding and the dedication of the most valuable resource - the staff. However, the insufficient resourcing of services running alongside the increase in public demand and expectation often fuelled by governmental statements can leave the practitioner in the impossible position of having to find yet more hours in the day to take on the extra demand. If agencies are to refocus the public services in a way that will truly work with families to prevent the risk of a child being abused, and are to avoid losing sight of those children who are at risk in the here and now, then a considerable amount of work is yet to be done.

The government has stated its intention to refocus services, including health, on the most vulnerable children and their families - vulnerable in the sense of being in need, an aspect of which could be in need of protection. In addition, the government has expressed its intention of making the welfare of children a community responsibility as well as the legal and ethical responsibility of the various public services concerned. This intention is one to be welcomed if it is what it would suggest, i.e. a complete reorganisation of the focus of the public services in such a way as to allow prevention to be the majority of work undertaken with the more urgent responsive work being in the minority by virtue of prevention. However, if this is to be achieved the reorganisation required would be immense, involving policy, funding arrangements, re-education and retraining of staff. Currently the structure of the public services make 'working together' often difficult as the various agencies seek to achieve their individual targets causing them to focus inwards rather than outwards. The government has put much store in the role of the primary healthcare team, the focus on the wellbeing of the community and the closer working relationship between community- and hospital-based staff and services. If this is to be achieved, effective community-based initiatives must be established in a consistent and systematic way across the country to prevent a system of 'care by geography' from developing. The balance between the appropriate level of government guidance and the need for flexibility to take into account local need is a tricky one, but one which must be achieved. However, before this refocusing occurs there must be established an interagency understanding of the meaning of a child in need, what those needs are, how best to address those needs and who will do what. Without this the risk is the appearance of a preventative service but one which is only 'skin deep', presenting a greater risk to children than the current often fragmented service that they currently receive. Bearing in mind that all children and families are involved with the NHS throughout their lives the importance of the healthcare practitioner in the refocusing debate is not to be underestimated. Arguably, it is they who know more about the wellbeing of children in all the dimensions that childhood entails than any of the other services they work with.

Domestic violence

It can be drawn from the case study linking Chapters 6, 7 and 8 that domestic violence is an often unseen and pervasive threat to children that can result in significant harm to their social, psychological and emotional development. Here it is important briefly to explore some of the issues, focusing on the effects that domestic violence had on the woman in the case study.

In the environment of a family where rules and expectations are often unclear and unspoken, the victim is at constant risk of transgressing a rule and thus incurring the anger of the perpetrator. This can trigger verbal abuse which may or may not escalate into violence. This causes the victim to behave in a manner aimed at minimising the potential of triggering the perpetrator's anger which, if unsuccessful, can result in her feeling responsible for her own assault. The verbal assault which may or may not lead to violence can cause the victim to experience constant anxiety, loss of self-confidence and self-worth, undermine her decision-making ability and her ability to protect herself and her children. Should the situation progress to physical violence, the victim, as well as being physically injured, is likely to experience further psychological assault from the feelings she has of being responsible for her own victimisation and her powerless state in relation the perpetrator.

Taking into account that domestic violence does not happen in a vacuum but more in an environment where the victim is repeatedly told she is unattractive, frigid, a poor mother etc. makes it almost impossible for her to retain the sense of self-worth required to either make a complaint to the police or leave the family home. Another factor which adds to this is the often real fear of retaliatory violence and possibly death as a result. Thus, to expect a woman to give an accurate account of how she sustained her injuries is in fact asking what, to her, may be the impossible. In order to do so she would have to acknowledge to herself her failure to prevent the assault and to risk greater injuries in the future. In addition is the expectation that as a mother she is responsible for the protection and wellbeing of her children - for the victim of domestic violence this can be seen as another example of her lack of self-worth and value as she sees herself failing once again. In addition she may see her only option of protecting her children from the perpetrator as allowing him to assault her rather than the children. In many situations the perpetrator will use the children's behaviour as justification for verbally and physically abusing the victim for her failure to control her children in the first place.

Sharing information of concern in the absence of a conviction

There is endless debate here about the potential risk to children and natural justice/civil liberties. From the practitioner's perspective the convicted offender, particularly the sex offender, feels like the tip of the iceberg, with those who are convicted forming the tip, and those who are known about but unconvicted forming the bulk.

There are proposals to develop interagency risk management and potentially dangerous offender's conferences where levels of risk to the community can be assessed and a plan produced to manage that risk best. In some areas this approach has been used for those individuals who are unconvicted but for whom practitioners have considerable concern at the risk they are posing to children. However, fears of libel and confusion over when it is justifiable to share confidential information, especially for those services whose primary client is the adult, child or young person causing that concern, has inhibited the sharing of vital information which, with hindsight, could have reduced and or minimised the abuse of a child.

There are no easy solutions to this dilemma, but we should remind ourselves that the majority of those who sexually abuse children do so in the absence of any conviction. Unless this area of debate is clarified with the interests of children in mind, practitioners could be at risk of being in the somewhat paradoxical position of protecting the rights of one group in society to abuse another.

Glossary of terms

The following terms are those which are often used in relation to children under child protection procedures and the definitions given here are both those most commonly in use and the ones used throughout this book.

Abuse Any experience of a child which undermines his or her health, development and wellbeing.

Accommodation Every local authority shall make provision for the reception and accommodation of children who are removed or kept away from home under Part V of the Children Act 1989.

Adoption The total transfer of parental responsibility from the child's natural parents to the adopter(s).

Affidavit A sworn written statement for use as Judicial proof.

Agency This term is used to represent both public and voluntary bodies.

Appeal 1 An appeal in care proceedings is heard by the High Court or, where applicable, by the Court of Appeal. All parties to the proceedings will have equal rights of appeal. On hearing an appeal, the High Court can make such orders as may be necessary to give effect to its decision.
2 Some ACPCs have established systems by which parents can appeal against being or not being placed on the child protection register. These systems of appeal are internal to each authority and not regulated by the Act.

Area Child Protection Committee (ACPC) In every local authority there is a need for a close working relationship between social service departments, the police service, medical practitioners, community health workers, the education service and others who share a common aim to protect the child at risk. Cooperation at the individual case level needs to be supported by joint agency and management policies for child protection consistent with their policies and plans for related service provision. There needs to be a recognised joint forum for developing, monitoring and reviewing child protection policies. This forum is the ACPC.

Assessment Almost any piece of work that looks at the needs of the child in a situation where risks may exist. See also comprehensive assessment.

Authorised person In relation to care and supervision proceedings, a person other than the local authority, authorised by the Secretary of State, to bring proceedings under S.31 of the Act. This covers the NSPCC and its officers. Elsewhere in the Act there is reference to persons who are authorised to carry out specified functions, e.g. to enter and inspect independent schools.

Care order An order made by the court under S.31(1)(a) of the Act placing the child in the care of the designated local authority. A care order includes an interim care order except where express provision to the contrary is made (S.31(11)).

Child By S.105(1) a person under the age of 18, except for certain financial purposes in Schedule 1 of the Children Act (not to be confused with Schedule 1 offenders; see below).

Child assessment order Section 43(1) of the Children Act 1989 provides that:

> On the application of a Local Authority or authorised person for an order be made under this section with respect to a child the court may make the order if, but only if, it is satisfied that:
> a) the applicant has reasonable cause to suspect that the child is suffering or is likely to suffer, significant harm
> b) an assessment of the state of the child's health or development or of the way in which he has been treated is required to enable the applicant to determine whether or not the child is likely to significant harm and
> c) it is unlikely that such an assessment will be made, or be satisfactory in the absence of an order under this section.

Child centred A term used to describe the need for all work in child protection to be undertaken in accordance with the child's needs.

Child in need A child, i.e. a person under 18 (s 105 (I)), is defined as being in need if he is unlikely to achieve or maintain, or to have the opportunity of achieving or maintaining, a reasonable standard of health or development without the provision for him of services by the local authority under Part III, or his health or development is likely to be significantly impaired or further impaired, without the provision for him of such services, or if he is disabled (S.17(10))

Child living away from home This is a complex description as children may live away from home in many circumstances. It is used here to describe a child being accommodated by the local authority.

Childminder A childminder may look after pre-school-age children. The regulations relating to childminding can be found in the HMSO publication *The Children Act 1989: Guidance and Regulations Volume 2. Day Care and Educational Provision for Young Children* (DoH 1991a).

Child protection plan This is the interagency plan identified once a child's name is recorded on the child protection register. It clarifies the roles and responsibilities of the practitioners involved with the family. The objective of the plan is to remove or minimise the risk to the child.

Child protection register In each area covered by a social services department, a central register must be maintained which lists all the children in the area who are considered to be suffering from or likely to suffer from significant harm and for whom there is a child protection plan.

Complaints procedure The NHS and social services are required to have a complaints procedure under the NHS & Community Care Act 1990 and The Children Act 1989.

Comprehensive assessment A complex and skilled process of gathering together and evaluating information about a child, his family and circumstances. Its purpose is to determine the child's needs in order to plan for his or her immediate and long-term care, and decide what services must be provided. Childcare assessments are usually coordinated by social services, but depend upon teamwork with other agencies. The NSPCC will often provide personnel to perform these assessments. Detailed information about conducting comprehensive assessments is provided in *Protecting Children: A Guide for Social Workers Undertaking a Comprehensive Assessment* (DoH 1991b).

Consent One of the responsibilities of a parent in relation to, e.g. the medical treatment of a child. If the child is capable of making an informed decision, his or her consent is required.

Contact The child's right to have contact with his/her parents. This replaces 'access', which was the parents' right to have access to their child.

Contact order Either an order under S.8 requiring the person with whom the child lives, or is to live, to allow the child to visit or stay with the person named in the order, or for that person and the child otherwise to have contact with each other or an order under S.34 where the child is in care for contact with a specified person.

Core group The small group of practitioners who work with the family when a child's name is recorded on the child protection register. They are responsible for various aspects of the child protection plan and will always consist of the key worker, often the health visitor/school nurse, and others as necessary.

Day care A person provides day care if he/she looks after one or more children under the age of eight on non-domestic premises for more than two hours a day (S.71).

Directions hearing This is a court hearing where the timetable of how the case will be managed within the court system is set out. The purpose of this is to reduce delay as much as is possible (see also timetable).

Disabled A child is disabled if he is blind, deaf or dumb or suffering from a mental disorder of any kind or is substantially or permanently handicapped by illness, injury or congenital deformity or such other disability as may be prescribed (S.17(11)).

Disclosure This is the description given to the defendant of the right to be given a copy of the evidence held against him or her by the prosecution.

Duty to investigate This is the duty placed on the local authority by the Act to investigate any situation where they feel a child in their area is suffering from or likely to suffer from significant harm.

Educational psychologist A psychologist who is specially trained in the branch of psychology that deals with the principles and methods of training and education in general.

Education welfare officer (EWO) A social worker with additional training in education who works with vulnerable school age children. This can include those at risk of truanting exclusion and/or abuse.

Emergency protection order (EPO) An order which a court can make for up to eight days (with an extension for a further seven days) if the court is satisfied that there is reasonable cause to believe that a child is likely to suffer significant harm if he is not removed to or does not remain in a place where he is being accommodated.

Empowerment A term used to describe the process by which practitioners work with parents and the child to help them to minimise or reduce the risk to the child both in the immediate period and long term.

Evidence Information that complies with the rules of evidence upon which a court will make its decision. In general, matters which are considered to be 'evidential' are matters of fact.

Family resource centre (FRC) Most social services will either have a family resource centre, or something similar to provide ongoing work with children and families.

Family panel Part of a division of the High Court created by the administration of the Justice Act 1970.

Family proceedings These are defined in S.8(3) as any proceedings under the inherent jurisdiction of the High Court in relation to children; and under Parts I, II, and IV of the Act, the Matrimonial Causes Act 1973, the Domestic Violence and Matrimonial Proceedings Act 1996, the Adoption Act 1976, the Domestic Proceeding and Magistrates' Courts Act 1978, S.1 and S.9 of the Matrimonial Homes Act 1983, and Part III of the Matrimonial and Family Proceedings Act 1984. It is important to note here those proceedings under Part V of the Children Act 1989, i.e. orders for the protection of children, are not family proceedings.

Family proceedings court All matters relating to children and families (unless criminal) will be dealt with by the family proceedings court.

Foster carer A person appointed by the local authority in accordance with The Foster Placement (Children) Regulations 1991.

***Guardian ad litem* (GAL)** A person, usually a social worker or other similarly trained individual, appointed by the court to look after the interests of children under the age of 17 when involved in court proceedings. They are independent of all parties concerned.

Harm Used to describe any experience of a child which undermines or potentially undermines his or her health or wellbeing.

In care A child who is accommodated by the local authority - this can be with foster parents or in a children's home or supported lodgings.

Independent schools All schools outside the control of the local education authority, and elsewhere called private or public schools.

Independent visitor An individual with an interest in the wellbeing of children who visits and befriends children who are accommodated. These individuals are carefully screened by the local authority and provide children with support and representation.

Initial child protection conference An initial child protection conference should be convened only after an investigation under Section 47 of the Children Act 1989 has been made into the incident or suspicion of abuse which has been referred to them. It should take place within eight working days, except where there are particular reasons for delay. It brings together family members, the child if appropriate and practitioners involved in order to make the interagency decision as to the level of risk facing the child and whether that level is sufficient to be described as significant harm. If so the child's name is recorded on the child protection register.

Injunction An order or a decree by which a party to an action is required to do or refrain from doing a particular thing.

Interagency A number of agencies sharing concern and responsibility for matters.

Interagency plan The interagency plan identified following the registration of a child's name on the child protection register. The plan will clarify the risks to the child and areas of the child's care which need improvement in order for the risk to be reduced or removed sufficiently to removed the child's name from the child protection register.

Interim care order An interim care order may be made for up to eight weeks, followed by extensions of a further four weeks at a time. The interim order gives the local authority parental responsibility while it further investigates, conducts assessments and develops the plan for the child.

Investigation The process by which social services investigate a referral from any source which suggests that a child living in their area is suffering or likely to be suffering from significant harm. This is sometimes referred to as a Section 47 investigation.

Joint interview The interview of a child by a specifically trained police officer and social worker undertaken in accordance with the publication The Memorandum of Good Practice (Home Office/DoH 1992). It is video recorded in order to avoid a child having to give evidence in court if possible.

Judicial review A uniform system for the exercise by the High Court of its supervisory jurisdiction over inferior courts, tribunals and public bodies.

Keyworker The practitioner, usually a social worker, assigned to a family as a result of the child's name being recorded on the child protection register. It is the key worker who has the role of coordinating the interagency child protection plan.

Legal aid A system governed by the Legal Aid Act 1988 by which a person can apply for financial assistance when involved with legal proceedings.

Local authority The middle tier of government sitting between Parliament and borough councils, with the power invested in it to establish and administer services such as social services and education. County councils, unitary authorities and metropolitan boroughs are all local authorities.

Looked after The term used to describe a child or young person who is accommodated by the local authority.

Paramountcy principle The principle which underpins the Children Act 1989 which states that in all activities the interests of the child must be the first and deciding factor of any action taken.

Parent Either the mother of the child, the father if married to the mother at the time of the child's birth or anyone who has been awarded parental responsibility by a court (see below).

Parental responsibility A key theme of the Act and defined as 'all the rights, duties, powers, responsibilities and authority which by law a parent of a child has in relation to the child and his property' (S.3(1)). Parental responsibility can be exercised by persons who are not the child's biological parents and can be shared among a number of persons. It can be acquired by agreement or court order.

Parties Parties to proceedings are entitled to attend the hearing, present their case and examine witnesses. The child is automatically a party to the care proceedings and the court will appoint a *guardian ad litem* and a solicitor to represent the interests of the child. Anyone with parental responsibility and the local authority will also each be a party and others may be able to acquire party status. A person with party status will be entitled to legal aid and to appeal against the decision of the court.

Partnership A principle of the Children Act 1989 which states that whenever possible practitioners should work in partnership with parents to help them to protect their children. It can also be extended to the idea that agencies should work together for the benefit of the child.

Permanency This refers to the child's right to stability of care, and presumes that intervention is either aimed at settling the child as quickly as is reasonable within the birth family or elsewhere, possibly through adoption.

Police protection Any police officer who has reasonable cause to believe that a child would otherwise be likely to suffer significant harm may remove the child to suitable accommodation and keep him there for up to 72 hours or ensure that he is not removed from hospital or any other place.

Practitioner This term has been used to describe those employed within in the statutory agencies.

Prohibited steps order An order that no step which could be taken by a parent in meeting his parental responsibility for a child, and which is of a kind specified in the order, shall be taken by any person without the consent of the prior court.

Recovery order An order that empowers the holder to remove a child from where he is living.

Refuge A dwelling run by the local authority or voluntary body which provides emergency, temporary accommodation for women and their children.

Rehabilitation After a significant period of separation from his natural parent or parents the child may be returned. Both the child and parent(s) should be supported through this process.

Residence order An order that states who the child is to live with.

Residential social worker A social worker who works with children who are accommodated in a local authority children's home.

Respite care Temporary, voluntary accommodation arranged by social services with a member of the wider family or foster parent apart from the parent or parents, to give an opportunity to resolve a crisis, to allow for a period of reconciliation or rest and recuperation.

Responsible person This is in relation to a supervised child and is 'any person who has parental responsibility for the child, any other person with whom the child is living'. With their consent the responsible person can be obliged to comply with certain obligations (S.3, paras 1 and 3).

Review child protection conference Once a child's name has been recorded on the child protection register at an initial child protection conference, there has to be a review child protection conference at the most six months later. This will continue for as long as the child's name remains on the register. An exceptions to this is if the child moves permanently to another social services area in which case a review child protection conference will be convened and the child's name removed. The area to which the child moves will convene a child protection conference and decide if the child's name is to be recorded on their child protection register.

Rules Rules of Court made by the Lord Chancellor which lay down the procedural rules which govern the operation of the courts under the Children Act 1989.

Schedule 1 Not to be confused with Schedule 1 of the Children Act 1989, but rather a term used to describe an offender with a criminal record including an offence against a child: 'He is a Schedule 1 offender'. Schedule 1 offences need not be of a sexual nature and can be committed by another child on a child and were originally listed in the 1933 Sexual Offences Act. The Schedule 1 label will remain with the offender for life.

Section 8 orders These are the orders that can be sought under Section 8 of the Children Act 1989.

Secure accommodation A court may make an order that a child is to be detained in local authority secure accommodation as a result of the sentence of the court or if sufficient concerns exist that not to do so would put the child at risk. These orders apply to children over the age of 13 years. If under 13 years, permission must be sought from the Secretary of State in advance.

Significant harm The criteria that must be reached before a child's name is recorded on the child protection register.

Socialisation A process by which children aquire the ability to see themselves as separate from their main carers and the position they occupy within the social environment. Socialisation is often divided into primary and secondary. Primary socialisation occurs in the first few years of life and develops from the home environment. Secondary is often used to describe the process once the child stars school and begins to accommodate the social world outside the home.

Specific issue order A court order giving directions for the purpose of determining a specific question which has arisen, or which may arise, in connection with any aspect of parental responsibility for a child.

Supervision order An order under S.3(1)(b) and including, except where express contrary provision is made, an interim supervision order under S.38.

Threshold The level of significant harm to a child that must exist or be thought to exist in order to record a child's name on the child protection register. This is a matter of judgement by those practitioners who attend the child protection conference.

Timetables Under the Act the court, in order to avoid delay because it is harmful to the child, has the power to draw up a timetable and give directions for the conduct of the case in any proceedings in which the making of a Section 8 order arises, and in applications for care and supervision orders (S.11 and S.32). For instance, the court may set dates by which certain evidence has to be lodged (see also directions hearing).

Ward of court A child who, as the subject of wardship proceedings, is under the protection of the High Court. No important decision can be made with regard to the child while he is a ward of the court without the consent of the wardship court.

Wardship proceedings The processes that relate to the wardship court.

Welfare checklist The list of factors that a court must ensure it takes into account when making any decision in relation to children. This does not apply in certain criminal offences committed by the child.

References

Ammerman R, Herson M (1990) Treatment of Family Violence: A Source Book. Wiley, New York.

Aries, P (1962) Centuries of Childhood. London, Jonathan Cape.

Bainham A, Cretney S (1993) Children and the Modern Law. Jordan Publishing, Bristol.

Bridge Child Care Consultancy (1995) Paul: Death by Neglect. Bridge Child Care Consultancy (on behalf of Islington ACPC), London.

Brown K, Davies C, Stratton P (1988) Early Predictions of Child Abuse. Wiley, Chichester.

Dale P, Davies M, Morrison T, Walters J (1986) Dangerous Families. Routledge, London.

de Bracton H (c. 1260) On the Laws and Customs of England. The University of Montana School of Law. http://grizzly.umt.edu.

Department of Health (1990) Child Abuse: A Study of Enquiry Reports 1980-1989. HMSO, London.

Department of Health (1991a) The Children Act 1989: Guidance and Regulations Volume 2. Day Care and Educational Provision for Young Children. HMSO, London.

Department of Health (1991b) Protecting Children: A Guide for Social Workers Undertaking a Comprehensive Assessment. HMSO, London.

Department of Health (1991c) Welfare of Children and Young People in Hospital. HMSO, London.

Department of Health (1991d) Working Together Under the Children Act 1989. HMSO, London.

Department of Health (1993) Child Protection: Medical Responsibilities. Guidance for Doctors Working with Child Protection Agencies. (Addendum to Working Together Under the Children Act 1989). HMSO, London.

Department of Health (1995) The Challenge of Partnership in Child Protection: Practice Guide. HMSO, London.

Department of Health (1995a) Child Protection: Clarification of Arrangements Between the NHS and Other Agencies. HMSO, London.

Department of Health (1995b) Child Protection: Messages from Research. HMSO, London.

Department of Health (1996) The Protection and Use of Patient Information. HMSO, London.

Department of Health (1997) Child Protection: Guidance for Senior Nurses, Health Visitors and Midwives. HMSO, London.

Department of Health (1998) The New NHS: Modern, Dependable. A National Framework for Assessing Performance. HMSO, London.

Department of Health (1998a) Our Healthier Nation. Green Paper. HMSO, London.

Department of Health (1998b) Working Together to Safeguard Children. Consultation Document. HMSO, London.

Department of Education (1988) Working Together for the Protection of Children from Abuse: Procedures Within the Educational Service, Circular No 4/88. HMSO, London.

Diamond B (1990) Legal Aspects of Nursing. Prentice Hall, New York.

Dickens C (1987) Hard Times. Oxford University Press, Oxford.

Engels F (1993) The Condition of the Working Class in England. Oxford University Press, Oxford.

Finkelhor D (1994) Child Sexual Abuse: New Theory and Research. Free Press Publishers, New York.

Frude N (1993) Understanding Family Problems: A Psychological Approach. Wiley, New York.

Hale M (1993 [1736]) History of the places of the Crown. In J Spencer, R Flin (eds) Evidence of Children: Law and Psychology, second edition. Blackstone, London.

Hibbert C (1987) The English: A Social History 1066-1945. HarperCollins, London.

Home Office (1989) The Piggot Report (Report of the Advisory Group on Video Recorded Evidence). HMSO, London.

Home Office (1998) Speaking Up for Justice. HMSO, London.

Home Office/Department of Health (1992) Memorandum of Good Practice. HMSO, London.

Humphries L (1997) Violence at home the prevention concept. Primary Health Care 7(1), 27-9.

Iwaniec D (1995) The Emotionally Abused and Neglected Child: Identification, Assessment and Intervention. Wiley, Chichester.

Jupp V (1993) Methods of Criminological Research. Routledge, London.

King M, Trowell J (1992) Child Welfare and the Law: The Limits of Legal Intervention. Sage, London.

L'Abate L (1994) Handbook of Developmental Family Psychology and Psychopathology. Wiley, New York.

Leach P (1990) Listening to Children. NSPCC/Longman, Harlow.

Masson J (1990) The Children Act 1989: Text and Commentary. Sweet & Maxwell, London.

Mitchels B, Prince A (1992). The Children Act and Medical Practice. Family Law Publishers, Bristol.

Moore B (1996) A Practitioners Guide to Predicting Harmful Behaviour, Whiting and Birch, London.

NHS Executive (1996) Child Health in the Community: A Guide to Good Practice. Department of Health, London.

O Hagan K (1992) Emotional and Psychological Abuse of Children. Open University Press, Buckinghamshire.

Rutherford L, Bone S (1993) Osbourne Concise Law Dictionary, eighth edition. Sweet & Maxwell, London.

Smith, JC, Hogan B (1992) Criminal Law, seventh edition. Butterworth, London.
Statt D (1990) The Concise Dictionary of Psychology. Routledge, London.
Wattram C (1992) Making a Case in Child Protection. Longman, Harlow.

Index